help!
WHY AM I
CHANGING?

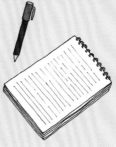

After studying English at the University of Oxford,
Susan Akass trained as a teacher and gained wide
experience in elementary schools, working mainly with 9–11
year olds and specializing in science. She has worked in the
UK and Australia, where she took a Master's degree in
Education at the University of Sydney. Her previous books
include *My First Book of My Body*, *My First Science Book*,
Bubbles and Balloons, and *Super Slime*. She is the general
editor of CICO Kidz "My First" series.

Consultants
Dr Frances Butcher (BMBS MA MSc MFPH)
Dr Rosanna Bevan (BSc BMBS MRCPCH)
James Hull (BA Hons PGCE)

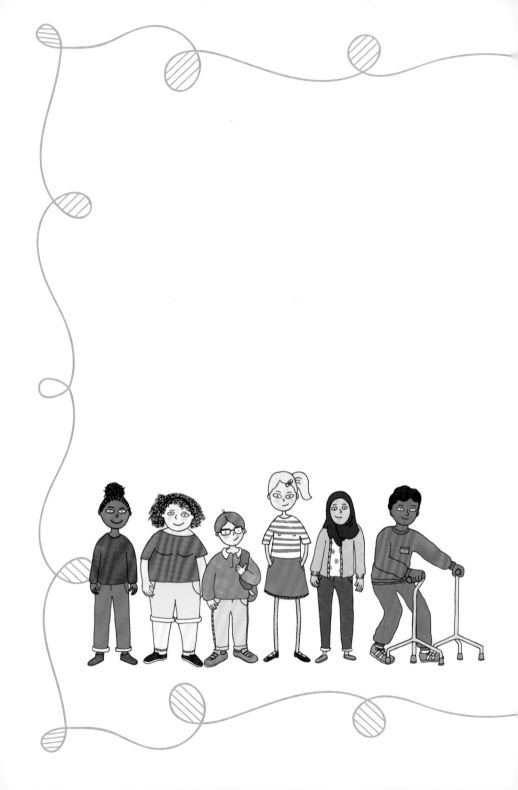

help!
WHY AM I CHANGING?

THE GROWING-UP GUIDE FOR PRE-TEEN BOYS AND GIRLS

SUSAN AKASS

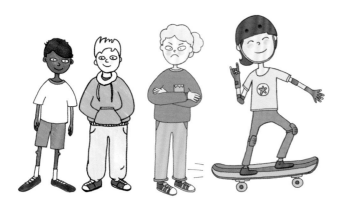

CICO **Kidz**
www.rylandpeters.com

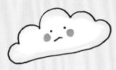

Published in 2019 by CICO Kidz
An imprint of Ryland Peters & Small Ltd
20–21 Jockey's Fields   341 E 116th St
London WC1R 4BW   New York, NY 10029

www.rylandpeters.com

10 9 8 7 6 5 4 3 2 1

ISBN: 978 1 78249 717 2

Printed in China

Editor: Caroline West
Designer: Louise Turpin
Illustrator: Jasmine Parker

In-house editor: Dawn Bates
In-house designer: Eliana Holder
Art director: Sally Powell
Production manager: Gordana Simakovic
Publishing manager: Penny Craig
Publisher: Cindy Richards

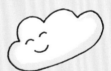

Note: Throughout the book, we have used the term
"parent" to denote a carer or any other person with
responsibility for looking after a child.

CONTENTS

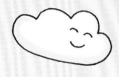

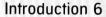

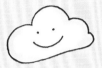

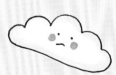

INTRODUCTION

In this book, you'll find the answers to questions that young people, like you, ask about puberty, which is the time when you begin to change from being a child to an adult. Puberty may already have begun for you, or it may still be some way off, but it will happen at some point in the next few years. It is an exciting time, but also a confusing one, when your body changes and so does the way you think and feel. It is a time when you have lots of questions, but may be too embarrassed to ask them.

Most sections of the book begin with a question and these questions are probably pretty close to the ones you want to ask. They are grouped into chapters. Chapter 1 deals with the changes in your body; Chapter 2 is all about how to care for your changing body; Chapter 3 is a chapter for girls, which answers some of the special questions they may need to ask, and Chapter 4 does the same for boys' questions (but you might want to read both chapters to find out about each other's worries and concerns); Chapter 5 is about the emotional challenges of puberty and how to care for your mind as well as your body; Chapter 6 is about coping at a time when you often feel self-conscious and unsure

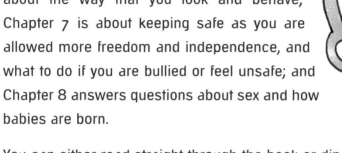

about the way that you look and behave; Chapter 7 is about keeping safe as you are allowed more freedom and independence, and what to do if you are bullied or feel unsafe; and Chapter 8 answers questions about sex and how babies are born.

You can either read straight through the book or dip into it when you need an answer to a question. And once you have some of the answers, I hope you will use them to start conversations with your parents, carers, or other adults who can give you more information, help, and advice. Talking about the worries that can arise during puberty is always the best way to deal with them. If you feel that you have no one to talk to, you could call one of the helplines listed on page 140.

I hope that all the questions you want to ask are covered somewhere in the book. If not, try looking on the websites also listed on pages 140–141.

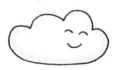

A MESSAGE TO PARENTS

Steering your children through puberty in the modern world is not easy. Puberty now starts at a much younger age for some children and ever-present media exposes them to ideas about sexuality, gender, and relationships much earlier than in the past. Pressures on modern children seem to be causing a surge of mental health problems, and allowing them greater independence can be a scary prospect.

This book is written for children aged 9 to 12 who are just entering puberty. It is much easier to talk to children of this age about what is going to happen in the next few years than it is to talk to teenagers who may think they know it all (and may well have got it all wrong).

It deals with the physical and emotional changes in puberty, discusses healthy living and safety, and introduces sex and relationships in a simple, straightforward way. However, please remember that this book is best used as a starting point for conversations and discussions in which you and your child can explore each subject further. These conversations can be difficult, but persevere because when your child keeps talking to you, it is both easier for you to cope with your changing child and easier for your child to get help if he or she needs it. Let your child know that you are happy to talk about the issues raised in the book.

I hope that reading this book might encourage children to open up about worries they are experiencing. If they need help for any physical or emotional problems, the advice given here is only a first step. Further help should be obtained from your child's teacher, your doctor, or other health professionals. The names of organizations that can give more detailed advice on issues raised are listed on pages 140–141. Some of these give very good guidance to parents about how to deal with the potential pitfalls of caring for children going through puberty.

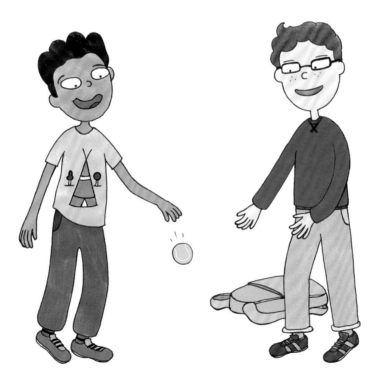

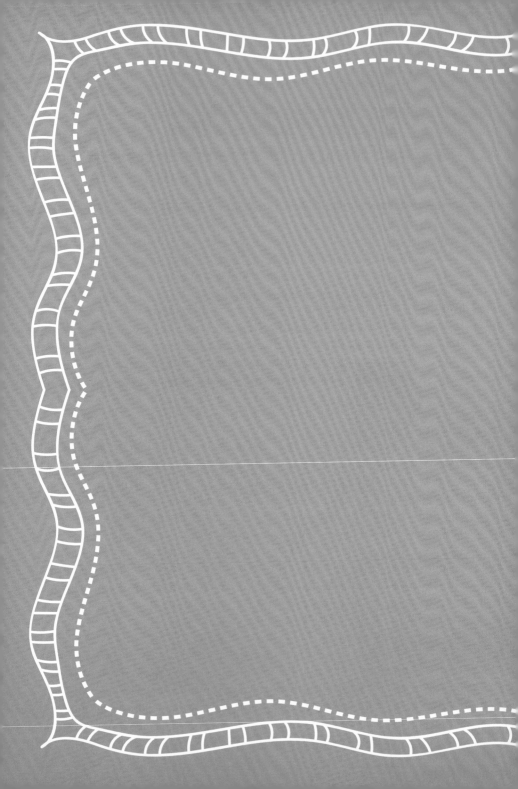

CHAPTER 1

GROWING UP

This chapter explains what is happening to you, or is about to happen to you, and why it happens. It gives you the details about how you will change as you go through puberty, both on the outside and on the inside. Some of the pictures may make you feel embarrassed, but try not to be! Find a quiet place to look and read, and discover all about the important bits of your body that don't get talked about much.

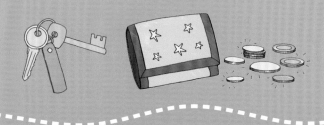

HOW HAVE YOU CHANGED SINCE YOU WERE BORN?

From the very first moment that you were born, you have been growing, changing, and learning, and you have learnt to do so many amazing things, but in the next few years you are going to grow, change, and learn a whole lot faster!

Can you find out the dates of your "milestones," like your first smile, first tooth, and first solid meal? Find some photos and videos of you when you were younger. Look for pictures you drew, stories you wrote, certificates you were awarded, and things your parents may have kept, such as your first pair of shoes. But be warned: parents are often great at keeping records for their first baby, but less good for second babies and any more that come along, because they are too busy by then!

Now think of all the things you have learnt to do since you were born. You've probably learnt to smile, crawl, stand, walk and run, talk, feed and wash yourself, use the bathroom, brush your teeth, dress yourself, swim, ride a bike, read, write, draw, use a computer, make friends, play sport, work as a team, take responsibility, clean your room (sometimes), and think for yourself. While you've been learning how to do all these things, your body has been changing. You've grown taller and stronger.

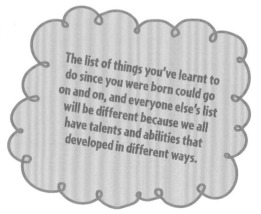

The list of things you've learnt to do since you were born could go on and on, and everyone else's list will be different because we all have talents and abilities that developed in different ways.

You have lost and gained teeth. Your hair has changed texture and maybe even color. Over the next few years you are going to change even more quickly as you go through puberty, which is the time when your body gradually changes from a child's to an adult's, so that one day, when you are fully grown up, you could have a baby of your own. Think about someone you know who is in their late teens (and the same sex as you), and play spot the difference. That will help you think about how you're going to change.

Puberty usually begins between age 8 and 13 in girls, and 9 and 14 in boys. You can't decide when it is going to start and it may happen to your friends at very different times. Don't worry if you've started puberty and your friends haven't, or if they have and you haven't. All children turn into adults at the time that is right for their bodies.

Puberty is an exciting time, but also a bit scary. In the next few years, as your body develops, you'll move schools, make new friends, learn new subjects, and become more independent. It is a time of up-and-down emotions and, above all, a time for lots of questions about what is happening.

From taking your first steps as a toddler to running around playing sports when you're older, you are constantly growing and changing.

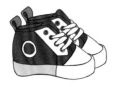 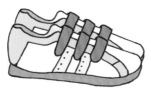 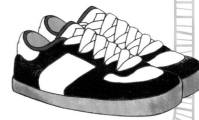

WHAT HAPPENS NEXT: TOWARD THE WORLD OF ADULTS

The changes that happen to you during puberty are all to do with getting your body ready for the day when you may decide to have a baby. A girl will become an adult woman who can get pregnant; a boy will become an adult man who can become a father. But becoming an adult is much more than being able to have a baby.

Being an adult is about taking responsibility for yourself and your actions. These are some of the ways in which you will learn to be an adult:

INDEPENDENCE: There will no longer be someone looking out for you all the time. When you go to high school you'll need to be organized about your schoolwork and possessions. You'll also have to think about being safe and responsible as you travel to and from school, go out with friends on your own, or stay home alone.

RELATIONSHIPS: You will meet more people, make new friends, start to have girlfriends or boyfriends (or both), and deal with different adults. To get on well with people, you will need to think about how you behave toward them and try to understand how they are feeling and thinking.

BEHAVIOR: Teenagers want to be cool. Sometimes being cool results in them getting into trouble, or hurting themselves or other people. Being an adult means knowing when to say "no" to things that you know are wrong and being brave enough to stick to your decision.

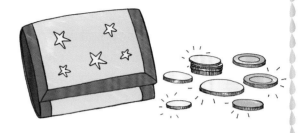

MONEY: As a teenager you may get a job, so you can have money of your own. You'll need to decide how you want to spend it, on what you need as well as on what you want. If you're going to be paid, you'll have to get to work on time, be polite and cooperative, look clean and tidy, and do your job efficiently.

CAREER: First jobs are usually just for pocket money. If you want to end up in your dream job, you'll need to work out what it is you want to do and how to prepare for it in a very competitive world. There will be exams to pass and experience to be gained. Only you can make it happen.

POLITICS AND SOCIETY: At 18 you can vote in an election. To know what to vote for you need to begin to understand the society you live in by watching or reading the news. Even before you can vote, you can campaign for a cause you believe in or you could help others by doing voluntary work or raising money for charity.

HEALTH: As you become more independent, you can decide when and what you eat, what exercise you do, and how you take care of your body. Many people today are unhealthy because of unhealthy food choices and not exercising enough; you can take responsibility for keeping yourself healthy.

HOW WILL MY BODY CHANGE ON THE OUTSIDE?

In the center of your brain is a grape-sized area called the hypothalamus. One day, for reasons even scientists don't yet understand, the hypothalamus decides it is time for you to change from a child to an adult. It sends out a chemical messenger called a hormone, which begins to trigger all the changes that happen in puberty.

 ## How a girl's body changes

⭐ Your skin and hair will get oilier and you may get pimples (spots).

⭐ Your hands and feet will grow.

⭐ You will sweat more.

⭐ You will begin to grow hair under your arms. Most girls like to remove this hair, so you don't often see it (see page 62). You'll also grow hair between your legs (in your pubic area–see opposite).

⭐ The hair on your arms and legs may get stronger and darker. Again, some girls like to remove the hair from their legs.

⭐ Your breasts will begin to develop and you will start to wear a bra.

⭐ You will have a "growth spurt" and begin to get taller more quickly.

⭐ You will gradually get curvier. Your hips will get wider, which will make your waist seem smaller.

⭐ You will begin your periods (see page 54).

⭐ Your face will gradually change so that your features become more distinct. You will look grown-up.

HOW WILL I LOOK DIFFERENT?

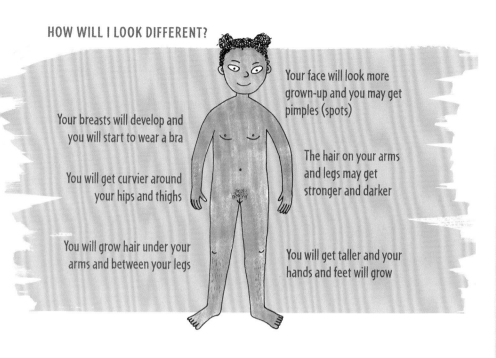

Your breasts will develop and you will start to wear a bra

You will get curvier around your hips and thighs

You will grow hair under your arms and between your legs

Your face will look more grown-up and you may get pimples (spots)

The hair on your arms and legs may get stronger and darker

You will get taller and your hands and feet will grow

WHAT ARE HORMONES?

Hormones are chemical messengers that travel in your bloodstream. For example, the hormone epinephrine (adrenaline) gives you extra energy to run away when you are in danger. In puberty, boys' testicles start producing other hormones, including testosterone, and girls' ovaries start making other hormones, including estrogen (oestrogen). These are behind all the changes at puberty.

How a boy's body changes

⭐ Your skin and hair will get oilier and you may get pimples (spots).

⭐ Your hands and feet will grow.

⭐ You will sweat more.

⭐ The hair on your arms and legs may get stronger and darker.

⭐ You will begin to grow hair under your arms and around your penis and testicles and later, maybe, on your chest and belly.

⭐ You will begin to grow hair on your chin and upper lip.

⭐ You will get taller, broader, and more muscular.

⭐ Your penis and testicles will get larger.

⭐ Your voice will get deeper.

⭐ Your face will gradually change so that your features become more distinct. You will look grown-up.

Did you know that when you start growing at puberty, your body grows in a particular order? Your hands and feet grow first, then your arms and legs. Your forearms lengthen before your upper arms, and your shin bones before your thigh bones. Next to grow is your spine; then boys will get a broader chest and shoulders and girls will get wider hips and pelvis. You grow so fast that your brain can't keep up and you may be more clumsy.

HOW WILL I LOOK DIFFERENT?

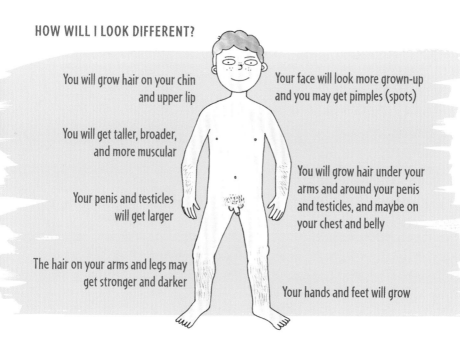

You will grow hair on your chin and upper lip

Your face will look more grown-up and you may get pimples (spots)

You will get taller, broader, and more muscular

You will grow hair under your arms and around your penis and testicles, and maybe on your chest and belly

Your penis and testicles will get larger

The hair on your arms and legs may get stronger and darker

Your hands and feet will grow

GIRLS: WHAT ARE MY SEX ORGANS?

At puberty, your body prepares for the time later in your life when you may want to have a baby. We go into detail about this later, but first you need to understand more about your body. This involves thinking about your genitals (sex organs) as well as the organs inside your body.

Boys know a bit about their genitals because they include the penis and testicles, which they can see and touch. But girls' sex organs are hidden. Most young people find talking about their genitals embarrassing. It shouldn't be. They are just another part of your body. You'll find it easier to talk about your genitals if you learn their correct names (see page 18).

 Do girls have genitals outside their bodies?

Yes! They are just more hidden than boys' sex organs. The easiest way for girls to get to know their genitals is to use a small mirror. Find a private place, lie on your back with your legs bent and apart,

GIRLS' GENITALS

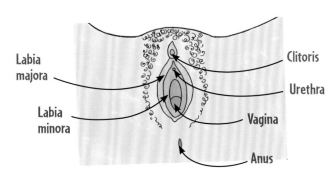

Labia majora — Clitoris

— Urethra

Labia minora — Vagina

— Anus

and hold the mirror between your legs. There are three openings (you may only be able to see two). There's a small hole at the front where your wee comes out (the urethra), but this is difficult to spot; a bigger one at the back where your poop comes out (anus); and the vagina in the middle. The vagina is a stretchy tube of muscles leading to an opening at the bottom of the uterus (womb). There are folds of skin around the vagina called labia. At the top of your genital area is a tiny bump called the clitoris, which can feel nice if you stroke it. The urethra, vagina, clitoris, and the labia are together known as the vulva.

 ## What organs are inside a girl's body?

Hold your fingertips and thumbs together to make a heart shape. Lower your hands so your fingertips are between your legs at the very top of the crack between your legs. The heart shows where your

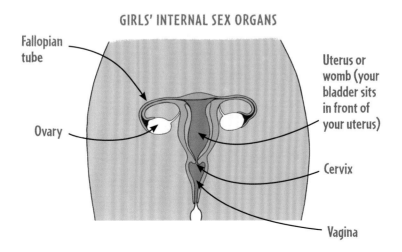

GIRLS' INTERNAL SEX ORGANS

Fallopian tube

Ovary

Uterus or womb (your bladder sits in front of your uterus)

Cervix

Vagina

> Ovaries produce a hormone (chemical messenger) called estrogen, which controls many of the changes that happen to girls in puberty, such as growing breasts and pubic hair.

uterus (womb) is inside your body. The womb is the place where a baby grows. You have two ovaries, one on each side of the womb. The ovaries are where the microscopic eggs, which are needed to make babies, are stored. Touch one of your first fingers to your thumb to make a circle. This is about the size of an ovary. Each ovary contains millions of eggs. The ovaries are attached to the womb by fallopian tubes. Your womb, fallopian tubes, and ovaries are your reproductive organs.

 How do my sex organs change at puberty?

Breasts are the first part of you to change. These are not really sex organs, but are linked to them because if you have a baby, your breasts will produce milk to feed him/her. Your breasts may begin to grow at any age from when you are around eight until you are in your teens. This is how it happens:

★ First you will notice that your chest isn't flat any more. Your nipples and areolae (the dark areas surrounding your nipples) are raised up on small bumps. Your nipples may hurt a bit sometimes.

★ Your nipples and areolae get darker and your breasts keep growing.

★ Your breasts, which might be a bit pointy at first, become rounder.

- ⭐ Your breasts can keep growing and changing right through your teens. The size and shape your breasts end up, and the color of your nipples and areolae, depend on your genes (see page 133). Nothing you do will make them grow faster or slower, or change shape.
- ⭐ You may grow a few hairs around the areolae.

 What does starting your periods mean?

> Starting periods can be a big deal for girls, but they are a sign that you're growing up and maturing, so should be seen as a special time and not something to worry about.

A period begins when one of the hormones (chemical messengers) in your blood tells your ovaries to get an egg ready to become a baby. This egg travels along one of the fallopian tubes toward your uterus (womb). At the same time, the womb gets ready for a baby by growing a thick lining. But to grow into a baby, the egg needs to be fertilized by a sperm (see page 131). If this doesn't happen, then the lining isn't needed, so it breaks away from the womb, comes down your vagina and out of your body onto your underwear, where you catch it on a sanitary napkin (pad) (see page 58). It looks just like blood. Periods last from 3–7 days, and will happen about once a month until you are around 50 years old.

We look at breasts and bras, as well as starting periods, in more detail in *Chapter 3: Girls and Puberty*.

BOYS: WHAT ARE MY SEX ORGANS?

Boys are used to seeing and touching their genitals because they hold their penis when they wee. Lots of little boys also use their penis like a security blanket and hold it when they are nervous or upset!

There are many, many nerves in the penis, which is why it feels nice to touch it. Under your penis are the testicles, which are inside a wrinkly bag of skin called the scrotum. Testicles produce the sperm needed to make babies (see page 130). The sperm is mixed with a fluid called semen that is produced in the prostate gland and two other glands called the seminal vesicles. A tube runs from the testicles to the prostate gland and out through the penis. This tube also has a branch leading to the bladder, so wee comes down it as well as sperm. A boy's anus is in the same place as a girl's, and is where poop comes out.

BOYS' INTERNAL SEX ORGANS

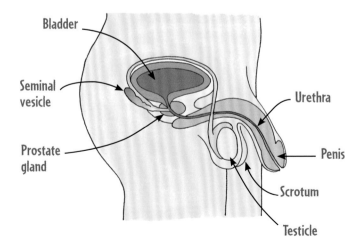

Bladder

Seminal vesicle

Prostate gland

Urethra

Penis

Scrotum

Testicle

How do my sex organs change at puberty?

You'll notice (and probably keep private) gradual changes to your penis and testicles. These are the changes that will happen. We look at some of them in more detail and explain how to deal with them in *Chapter 4: Boys and Puberty*.

⭐ First your testicles begin to grow. Your scrotum (the bag that holds your testicles) becomes larger, redder, and thinner-skinned, and hangs down lower. You get a few straight dark hairs around your penis.

⭐ Next your penis gets longer. You'll get more hair around it and the hairs begin to get curly. You may have been circumcised as a baby, which means the foreskin has been removed for religious, social, or health reasons. A circumcised penis looks different to an uncircumcised one.

⭐ Your testicles, scrotum, and penis keep growing. You penis also begins to get thicker. Your penis and testicles will carry on growing until your late teens.

⭐ You keep getting erections, which is when your penis becomes stiff and stands up. You will already know about erections because you started having them when you were a baby. They will happen more often in puberty.

⭐ Your testicles start to produce sperm (see page 130 to find out more about this).

BOYS' GENITALS

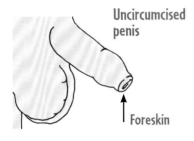

Uncircumcised penis

Foreskin

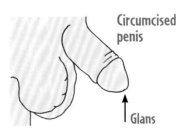

Circumcised penis

Glans

CHAPTER 2

CARING FOR YOUR BODY

As a little kid, showering was probably not high on your list of things to do, but that's about to change. When your body changes you have to look after it in new ways and this chapter tells you all you need to know about coping with everything from body odor (BO) to smelly feet and pimples (spots). It is also full of good advice about looking after yourself so that you grow up fit, healthy, and proud of your body.

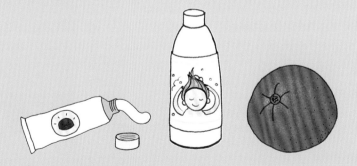

KEEPING CLEAN

During puberty you sweat more, your skin and hair become oilier, and you may get pimples (spots). Keeping yourself clean becomes extra important. Your parents may be amazed at how much time you begin to spend in the bathroom!

 I heard someone say that I've got BO. What should I do?

You can get body odor (BO) when bacteria, which live on the skin, break down sweat. All young people who are going through puberty sweat more and begin to get more smelly, so everyone needs to follow these simple rules:

⭐ Shower or wash well every day and after any activity when you have got hot and sweaty. That will kill off the bacteria.

⭐ Use a good antiperspirant or deodorant under your arms, which is the place where you get most BO. Antiperspirants actually stop the sweat glands under your arms from producing sweat. Deodorants kill off the bacteria that cause the smell. Both usually contain perfume which can mask any bad smells. Some of these products are stronger than others. For a while you might need to use a strong one.

⭐ Change your clothes every day, so they are not full of stale sweat which will go smelly. Some man-made fabrics can make you sweat more. Cotton is better, or you can wear modern "wicking" fabrics for sport and outdoor activities.

⭐ Don't forget to take your wash kit (and use it) when you stay away from home.

My hair has starting getting really oily. How often should I wash it?

At the base of each hair you have a tiny gland which produces an oily substance called sebum. This keeps your hair from drying out and becoming brittle, but in puberty you often get too much of it. To keep your hair looking good, wash it as often as you need to, probably every day or every two days. You may also need to give your hair an extra wash after sport, but this depends a bit on your hair type. If you wash and blow-dry fine hair too often, for example, it can get dry and brittle at the ends.

I think I've got dandruff. How can I get rid of it?

In puberty, you can get dandruff, as well as oily hair. Dandruff is white or gray flakes of skin which come from your scalp and catch in your hair or fall onto your shoulders. It is easy to treat with an anti-dandruff shampoo from your grocery store or pharmacy. If one type doesn't work for you, just try another. Start by using the shampoo every day. Once the dandruff has cleared up, you may then only need to use it once a week. If it gets worse and your scalp gets sore or itchy, see your doctor who can prescribe something stronger.

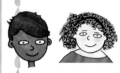

What can I do about my smelly feet?

Loads of young people get really smelly feet during puberty for the same reason that they get BO: sweat and bacteria (see page 28). Don't worry, as there are lots of things you can do to help.

⭐ Wash your feet with a strong antibacterial soap, which you can buy from pharmacies, twice a day for about a week to stop your feet smelling.

⭐ Get two pairs of shoes (if possible). If you wear the same shoes every day, they get damp with sweat and bacteria will breed in them. You need to let the shoes dry out before wearing them again, so swap them each day. This will be expensive if your feet are growing fast, but your family will be grateful to be rid of the smell. Make sure the shoes are made of breathable fabrics and are not all plastic.

⭐ Wash and dry your feet well every day and put on clean cotton socks (not nylon). Change your socks for sport. Go barefoot at home, but wash your feet first!

⭐ Spray your feet with an antiperspirant or deodorant. Just use the same one for your feet as you do under your arms.

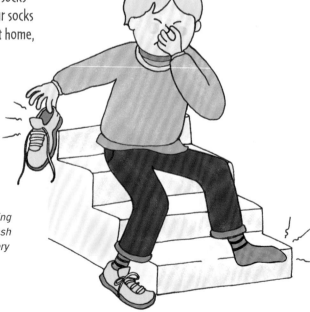

You may get smelly feet during puberty, so make sure to wash and dry them thoroughly every day. You'll need to change your socks daily too!

Someone said that I have bad breath. What should I do?

At your age many young people get cavities, gum disease, and bad breath. Bacteria are the problem again. To get rid of the bacteria which cause tooth decay, you need to brush your teeth twice a day with a soft toothbrush and use a good fluoride toothpaste. You should also learn to floss between your teeth or use interdental brushes (your dentist or hygienist will show you how). Try to avoid sugary drinks and snacks too, as these feed the bacteria which cause tooth decay and could destroy your perfect film-star smile. And make sure to see a dentist every six months. You will be given treatments to protect your teeth.

> When you were little, your parents made sure you brushed your teeth to keep them clean and your breath fresh. Now, with no one to nag, you may just forget. Bad move!

Should I brush my teeth differently if I have braces?

Yes, you need to be even more careful about cleaning your teeth and avoiding certain foods when you have braces (see page 93). Most dentists and orthodontists recommend brushing your teeth after each meal to get out food that may have caught on them. They may also tell you to use special brushes or flosses. Take notice of what they say because you don't want to have smelly breath or, at the end of your treatment, find your smile is spoiled by staining and tooth decay!

WASHING YOUR GENITALS

**Now it's back to those embarrassing bits which you don't like to talk about!
It is especially important that you keep your genitals clean because
they can get smelly and sometimes sore or itchy.**

 ### Girls: how should I wash down there?

You should wash your vulva (the whole area down there) daily, using warm water, and nothing else. Your vagina cleans itself naturally. It is also full of "good bacteria" which keep it healthy; soap or other products can harm these. If you've started your periods, it's even more important that you wash your genitals and keep them clean. If you are worried about getting blood on your towel, dry around your vagina with some toilet paper first, then use the towel and put your underwear back on. If you get smelly or itchy down there, tell a parent or a nurse or doctor.

Girls: I've been told I should wipe from front to back when I have a poop. Why is this?

Wiping from front to back keeps poo well away from your urethra (the hole you wee through). Poop is full of lots of nasty bacteria which can enter the urethra and travel to your bladder (where wee is collected). This can result in an infection that can make you feel really ill.

Boys: my penis is a bit smelly. How should I keep it clean?

You should wash your penis once a day in warm water. Don't use strong soap or shower gel, as these will make your penis sore. If you are not circumcised (see page 25), then pull the foreskin back gently and wash underneath it. If you don't do this, white cheesy stuff called smegma can collect underneath. Smegma is natural and keeps the head of the penis comfortable, but it can be a breeding ground for bacteria if you don't clean it out. Boys who are circumcised also need to wash their penises well. All boys should wash and dry carefully around their testicles and back to their anuses. This is a hot, sweaty, hairy area, with no air to dry it out, which means it can get smelly.

REMEMBER TO CHANGE YOUR UNDERWEAR
As well as washing your genitals every day, you should change your underwear daily, too. Girls, you can now buy period-proof underwear and swimwear if you've started your periods and don't always want to rely on sanitary napkins (pads) or tampons (see page 58 for more advice on sanitary wear).

DEALING WITH PIMPLES

Most young people get pimples (spots) at some stage during puberty. Girls tend to get them a bit younger than boys, starting between ages 10 and 13, but you are unlikely to get bad pimples until you are in your teens.

 My face is breaking out in pimples (spots). Why is this and is there a cream that will cure them?

Each hair follicle, or pore, in your skin contains a hair with a tiny gland at the base. These glands secrete an oily substance called sebum, which keeps your skin soft and waterproof. This is the same sebum that makes your hair oily. In puberty, you produce a lot more sebum, and the pores can get blocked with sebum and dead skin cells. This causes whiteheads just under the skin, blackheads if the pores are open to the air, and, if the pore gets infected with bacteria, red pimples, sometimes with a pus-filled yellow head.

Sometimes, you can get lots of pimples, a condition that is known as acne. This can make you very self-conscious. The important thing is to find a way of treating it that works for you. When your hormones settle down in your late teens you may well "grow out" of your acne.

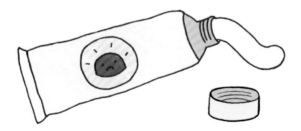

If you do get pimples, try the following to get rid of them:

⭐ Gently wash your face twice a day with mild soap and warm water. Don't scrub your face, as this can make pimples worse.

⭐ Try an "over-the-counter" pimple cream from your pharmacy. If this doesn't work, and your pimples get worse, see your doctor who will prescribe stronger treatments. Never put up with acne. It can always be treated, but you must follow the treatments carefully.

⭐ Try not to squeeze pimples and blackheads because this can cause infection and scars. If you're tempted to squeeze them (and most people do sometimes), wash your hands and face really well first and use a tissue.

⭐ Acne treatments can make your skin red and dry, so use a good moisturizer. Look for one that is labeled "non-comedogenic," which means it won't block your pores. The moisturizer should be light and oil-free. Don't use moisturizers that are greasy.

⭐ If you want to use makeup to cover pimples, use a tinted moisturizer which is non-oily and non-comedogenic (which means it won't block your pores). Some brands also contain salicylic acid, which is an acne treatment used to unblock pores, so they actually help your skin, too. Alternatively, use a cover stick/concealer to hide individual pimples.

⭐ Girls: if you've started your periods, remember that your pimples can get worse around the time your period is due.

Acne is caused by changes in your hormones and not by anything you eat. However, eating healthy food, drinking plenty of water, and getting lots of fresh air and exercise are all ways to help improve your skin.

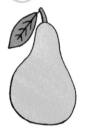
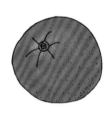
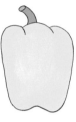

EAT WELL, GROW WELL

You need food to grow, and during puberty you do a lot of growing. You grow taller and even your brain grows. Boys get broader and gain lots of muscle, while girls get breasts and a softer figure with more body fat. To help you grow strong and healthy, at the right body weight, and with skin and hair in great condition, you need to eat the right food containing the right nutrients. Just as importantly, the food you eat now will set you up for a healthy adult life.

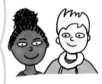

People say to eat a healthy diet. I bet that means giving up all the food I like best!

Hopefully not, but if the only food you like is "junk food" you should try to change the way you eat. The wrong foods are making too many children overweight, unhealthy, and unhappy. As you become more independent, you get to choose what you eat more often, so try to follow these rules as much as you can:

⭐ Eat regular meals, including breakfast.

⭐ Eat more fruit and vegetables (try for at least five a day).

⭐ Stick to healthy snacks (see Box, opposite).

⭐ Drink water or sometimes milk.

⭐ Keep junk food for occasional treats.

What are junk foods?

Junk foods are factory-made foods that contain lots of sugar, fat, and salt. They include candy, chocolate, ice cream, sugary breakfast cereals, chips (crisps), French fries (chips), cookies, cakes, pizzas, pies, fast foods like takeout burgers and fried chicken, sauces and salad dressings, sodas (fizzy drinks), and milkshakes. They are probably to blame for how overweight and unhealthy many people are getting and you should eat/drink less of them. But you don't need to give them up altogether. (Drink sugar-free soda, if you can.)

I hate vegetables and fruit. How can I ever eat my five a day?

Start by having fruit on your breakfast cereal. Have a handful of cherry tomatoes, carrot sticks, or cucumber sticks for lunch and fruit for

HEALTHY SNACKS

★ Fresh fruit

★ A handful of nuts (plain, not salted)

★ Vegetable sticks dipped in hummus

★ Whole-grain bread or toast, pita bread, bagels, crackers, rice cakes, oat cakes, soft pretzels, tortilla wraps, or popcorn (unsweetened). Have these with cheese, cream cheese, tuna, chicken, turkey, peanut butter, egg, hummus, tomato, or avocado

★ Sugar-free cereal with fruit or oatmeal (porridge) with raisins

dessert. Get your parents to hide vegetables in the food they cook. There are onions and canned tomatoes in spaghetti Bolognese, for example, and you could add vegetables like carrots or kidney beans. Try eating broccoli or peas; most young people learn to like them. Ask your parents to show you how to make a smoothie for dessert and add frozen spinach. It won't change the taste much, but it is really good for you. And why not learn to cook and make your own veggie creations?

I thought fruit was healthy, so why do people say not to drink fruit juice or eat too much dried fruit?

Fruit is healthy because it contains vitamins, minerals, and fiber (which is good for your guts), but it also contains sugar. A glass of fruit juice or a handful of dried fruits contain lots more sugar than one piece of fruit, so they are not so good for your weight or your teeth. Dried fruit also sticks to your teeth so is more likely to cause decay. It is fine to have a glass of fruit juice or a small smoothie as one of your five a day, but not more. A handful of dried fruit is also good, especially as part of a meal, but not too often.

Is my dad right that it's not healthy to be a vegetarian?

He's not right. Being vegetarian is very healthy if you eat lots of different vegetables, beans, and nuts. But if you only eat pizza, you may miss out on important nutrients. Lots of young people become vegetarian at your age because they begin to realize where meat comes from and don't like the way animals are treated.

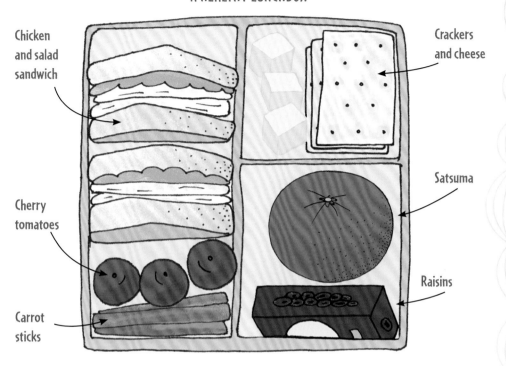

Chicken and salad sandwich

Crackers and cheese

Cherry tomatoes

Satsuma

Carrot sticks

Raisins

What should I say if my friends ask me to go on a diet with them?

If a doctor or nurse says you're overweight, they'll also advise you how to lose weight. Follow their advice, and get your family to help. If friends ask you to go on a diet with them be careful! Do you or they really need to lose weight or are they trying to look like a skinny celebrity? Many images of celebrities are airbrushed on a computer, so they don't really look like that. The "fad" diets they promote lack the nutrients you need and can stop you developing normally. The best way to look good is to eat healthier food and be more active (see page 40).

KEEP MOVING: HOW EXERCISE HELPS

Count how many hours you have spent sitting down today. It may surprise you. We all spend too much time sitting rather than being active, and it's not good for us. Young people your age should be fit and strong.

Being active is good for your brain, as well as your body. Exercise makes you learn better, feel happier, and sleep better. Being fit at your age will also affect your health when you're an adult, so it is really important. You should be active for at least an hour every day (see Box, opposite). Exercise can help you in these ways:

⭐ You get fitter, and grow and develop in a healthy way.

⭐ You have fun with other people.

⭐ You build a stronger heart, bones, and muscles.

⭐ Your concentration improves.

⭐ You do better at school.

⭐ You feel more confident.

⭐ Your posture and balance improves.

⭐ You sleep better.

⭐ You feel less worried and stressed.

Try to fit in the following three types of exercise each week:

AEROBIC: Anything that makes you out of breath and gets your heart and lungs working. You need lots of this.

STRENGTH BUILDING: This gives you strong bones and muscles. Crossing the monkey bars, tennis, skipping,

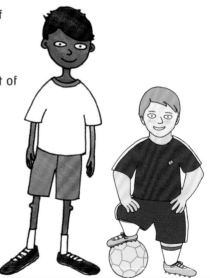

HOW TO FIT IN YOUR HOUR A DAY

*Walk or cycle to school, walk the dog, run, dance,
play sport, kick a ball, play tag, skateboard,
rollerblade, ice skate, climb trees, turn cartwheels, do
handstands, bounce on a trampoline, swim,
take up a martial art like judo or karate, go hiking
with your family, go surfing, do jobs
around the house (rake leaves, clean
the car, vacuum). And, as fresh air is
good for you, at least some of these
should take place outside!*

*It is easier to get enough
exercise if you make some
of it part of your daily routine,
such as walking or cycling
to school, or even just having
fun on your skateboard.*

push-ups, and climbing are all good
strength-building activities.

FLEXIBILITY: Young people are more flexible than
adults, but you will lose this flexibility if you don't keep
stretching. Warm-up stretches, dance, gymnastics, and
martial arts are all good for keeping you supple and flexible.

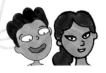 **I want to do more sport, but my friends don't want to. They just want to play computer games or watch DVDs**

All young people are told too much screen time is bad for them, but many don't want to know. If your friends don't want to be fit like you, then why not try out a new sport at a local club and make some new friends? There are all kinds of sports you can try, which you might not get to do at school. How about judo, fencing, trampolining, or cycling? If you are already keen on a sport at school, you could join a club where you will have more time and expert coaching to develop your skills. Go along to your local sports center and see what is on offer. Your old friends might decide it all sounds cool and join you.

I want to build up my muscles. How should I do it?

You may admire the bodies of men and women in movies or on TV, but you won't be able to build much muscle until you start puberty. That's when your body begins to produce the hormones needed to build muscle. But both boys and girls can still get fit and strong before puberty. Chin-ups, sit-ups, and push-ups are all great for your body if done properly; watch online instruction videos from a trusted source to find out how.

I hate sport, so how can I get fit?

Some young people love sport and are super-competitive, while others think they are useless and that nobody wants them on their team. If you don't like school sport, you need to find a sport or exercise that's right for you outside school. Think about what motivates you. Are you competitive or not? Would you prefer a team or individual sport? Would you enjoy focusing on something difficult (like rock climbing) or do you want something that's easy to start such as running or hiking. Some summer camps let you try different sports and you may find one that suits you. The more you do a sport, the more motivated and confident you'll become. Don't feel you have to be brilliant at it. Most people are not Olympic athletes or major league players. They just want to challenge themselves and have fun.

I'd like to do sport, but feel self-conscious about my body

If you are self-conscious about being overweight, or very skinny, or about your hairy legs or knobbly knees, school sport and PE lessons can be horrible. Other children can be cruel and sports teachers may be unsympathetic. Check out these tips and see if they help you:

⭐ For school sport and PE lessons, ask to wear a loose tracksuit (or leggings), which will cover you up more. A good teacher should be encouraging.

⭐ Look around you. Shot-putters at the Olympics, for example, are huge, but they're proud of their bodies, while people who run marathons come in all shapes and sizes.

⭐ Remember, the more you exercise and improve at an activity, the more confident you'll become about your body and that confidence will spread to other activities.

⭐ If you are overweight, you might like to think about finding a special class for overweight young people where you can encourage each other to get fit.

GETTING ENOUGH SLEEP AND REST

Scientists keep discovering more about how important sleep is and how much sleep you need. At your age, they say you should get 9 to 10 hours a night. So, if you have to get up for school at 7am, you need to be asleep by 9pm.

Some young people think it is cool and grown-up to stay up late. Of course, it's fine to stay up for a special occasion, but sleep is important for lots of different reasons, so it's not cool to stay up on school days. The changes to your hormones that happen in puberty are triggered when you are in deep sleep. During puberty, your brain is also reorganizing itself and it does this when you are asleep. If you don't get enough sleep, this is how it can affect your life:

★ You find it more difficult to think and learn. As a result, you may get lower grades at school.

★ Your reaction times are slower. You become less good at sport (and also computer games).

★ You are clumsier and more likely to get injured.

★ You are moody, unhappy, and get into arguments more easily.

★ You make more mistakes.

★ You grow more slowly.

★ You are more likely to get ill.

★ You are more likely to be overweight.

I can't get to sleep when I go to bed early. Does that mean I need less sleep?

Unfortunately not. It probably means you have got into a bad sleep habit. The following tips might help you sleep more easily:

★ Go to bed and get up at about the same time every day. Your brain learns when it's time to sleep. Don't sleep in too late at weekends, as this will upset your body clock. See page 46 for more advice on good sleep habits.

★ Keep your bedroom cool, quiet, and dark.

★ Have at least 1 hour of screen-free time before bed. Light from screens messes up the chemicals in your brain that make you fall asleep.

★ If you have a phone, leave it in the kitchen, so you are not tempted to look at it at night.

★ Being active during the day really helps, but do something calm just before you go to bed. Try reading or listening to an audiobook or podcast.

★ Don't eat a lot just before you go to bed, but don't go to bed hungry either. A small snack and a glass of milk can help you sleep. Avoid sodas (fizzy drinks) that contain caffeine.

★ Get your homework done before you go to bed, so you don't worry about it.

★ If you are anxious about something, try to talk it over with a parent before you go to bed. Or perhaps write it down in a journal.

If you can't sleep, tense each part of your body, then relax it. Start with your toes, screwing them up, then relaxing them. Move up through your legs, buttocks, and stomach. Go on to your fingers (hold them in a fist to tense), arms, jaw (clench teeth to tense), and eyes (scrunch up to tense). Follow your breathing in and out until you feel sleepy.

I find it really hard to get up for school in the mornings

You're not alone. Scientists have discovered that brain changes in puberty mean your body clock resets itself and you naturally want to go to bed later and sleep longer in the mornings. Some high schools (secondary schools) have even changed their starting times because students learn better if they start later. Maybe you should suggest this to your school council! To help avoid morning panics and arguments, get everything ready for school before you go to bed and set your alarm clock early enough to give yourself plenty of time to get going gradually. Kick off the duvet or try to jump straight out of bed when you wake up, so that you don't fall asleep again. Once you are up, you will gradually feel less sleepy and will start the day feeling much happier and calmer.

Set your alarm clock to give you lots of time to get ready for school in the morning.

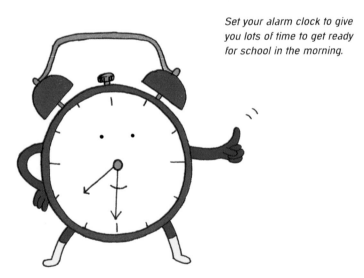

VISITING HEALTH PROFESSIONALS

At your age you should visit the dentist and optician for regular check-ups. There will also be times when you need to visit your doctor.

When you were younger your parents knew what was happening to your body. As you get older, you need to tell them if you have concerns, but you may feel embarrassed to talk about your body. Remember that your parents, and doctors and nurses, aren't embarrassed and only want to help. You can always choose to have a parent or other trusted adult with you when you see a doctor or nurse.

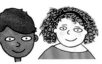

Why do I need special vaccinations?

Another reason to see a doctor is to complete your vaccinations. Most likely you will already have had a lot of vaccinations as a baby and small child to stop you getting ill. At puberty, some of these vaccinations need a booster and there are also new ones you should have. If you haven't had all your shots as a baby, talk this over with your parents or doctor. Vaccines are very safe and can prevent serious diseases. The age at which you get your shots varies from country to country, but it is important for all young people to have the following vaccinations:

⭐ The HPV vaccine when you're 12 or 13 because this can prevent some forms of cancer in later life.

⭐ Another shot of the meningococcal vaccine, which can prevent meningitis, a serious disease that is more common in teenagers and young adults.

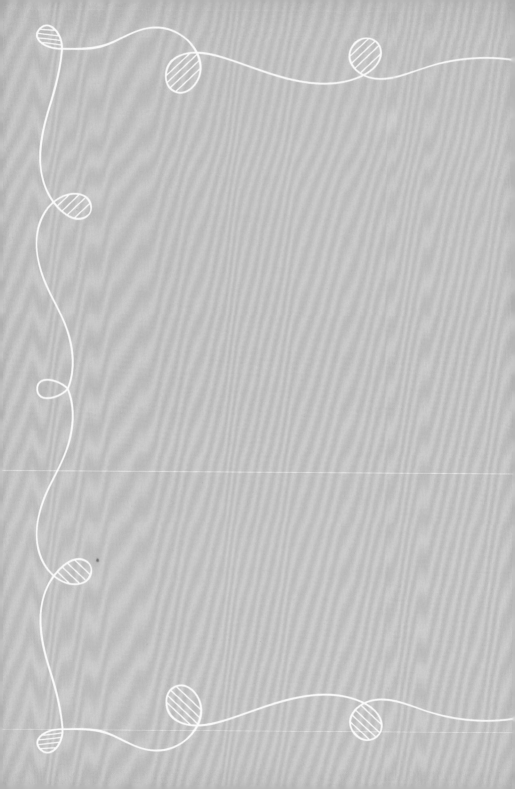

CHAPTER 3

GIRLS AND PUBERTY

Girls, this is a chapter for you (although boys may want to read it
too, so they know what's going on with their friends, classmates,
and sisters). It deals with some tricky subjects, starting with
breasts and bras, then continuing with a whole lot about periods
and, finally, a section about body hair and shaving. It will
get you ready for the big changes in your life as
you begin to leave your little girl self behind.

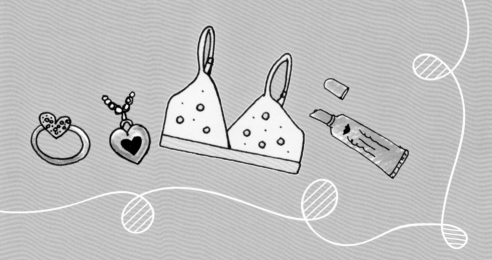

BREASTS, BRAS, AND OTHER BITS

Getting your first bra-style top is one of the first signs that you are no longer a little girl. Some girls can't wait to get one, while others would rather put it off. When you do decide to get one, there's plenty of choice.

When should I get a bra?

It is up to you when you get a bra. Just as some girls wear bikini tops on the beach even when they are flat-chested, so many begin to wear crop tops or bralettes before they need a bra. When your breasts are growing, wearing a crop top or bralette can help you feel less self-conscious about them. As your breasts get bigger, wearing a bra is usually more comfortable than going without. Bras stop your breasts bouncing and wobbling when you run, dance, or do sport!

How do I know what size to get?

The best way is to ask a parent to take you to a store which offers a measuring service. You need two measurements for a bra: one right around your back just below your breasts and one around the widest point of your breasts. The first measurement gives you your chest size and from the second you can work out your cup size. If you can't find a measuring service (or are a bit embarrassed),

Your bra should hold your breasts firmly. If you bulge out at the sides, the bra is too small. If the bra crinkles or sags open, then it's too big. Find one that is comfortable and suits your style.

measure your chest size and then try on a few bras with different cup sizes.

What type of bra should I get?

Many stores do a range of first bras designed for girls like you. These are often called trainer bras. Alternatively, you can get sports bras which are more like bralettes, but designed to hold you firmly to stop your breasts from bouncing. You will need at least three bras so that you can change them and wash them frequently.

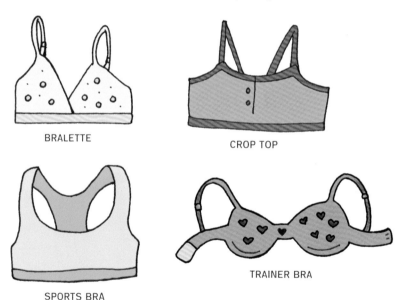

BRALETTE

CROP TOP

SPORTS BRA

TRAINER BRA

Trainer bras or crop tops are perfect when your breasts start to develop. Later you'll find a great choice of adult bras, bralettes, and sports bras. Some types will make your breasts look smaller; others make them look bigger. It's up to you which type you wear.

Why is one of my breasts bigger than the other?

Breasts are often different sizes when they first start growing and then they even out. One of your breasts may even begin to grow before the other. Sometimes they remain different sizes. Just like people have different-sized feet or different-colored eyes, so some women have different-sized breasts. But if you wear a good bra, you won't be able to tell.

Girls' breasts start growing at different ages, but everyone develops in their own time and so this is nothing to be concerned about.

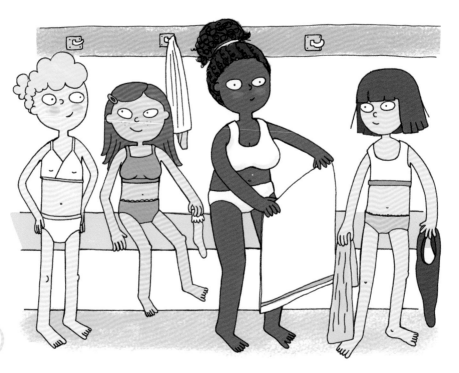

Why do my nipples point in?

Most women's nipples point out, but a lot of women's nipples point in. This is called having inverted nipples. It is nothing to worry about and you will still be able to breastfeed a baby (see page 134) just the same, if you wish to.

Why do my breasts sometimes feel sore?

Breasts can feel sore when they first begin to develop and also just before a period. It could also be that your breasts are growing and your bra is now too tight!

Is it wrong to touch myself down there?

If you look at the diagram on page 20, you will see that a clitoris is part of your genitals. Like a boy's penis, the clitoris is full of nerves and it feels good to touch it. Stroking or rubbing your clitoris is called masturbation and it isn't wrong. It is completely normal, although it is something you would always do in private. If you keep stroking, it feels nicer and nicer until the feeling reaches a peak called an orgasm, which is what can happen when you have sex. As you go through puberty, and begin to think more about sex, masturbation helps you learn what gives you sexual pleasure. Both girls and boys masturbate, girls by rubbing their clitorises, boys by rubbing their penises (see page 69).

WHAT HAPPENS WHEN I START MY PERIODS?

This is a long section because girls ask lots of questions about periods. Although periods may seem a bit worrying, remember that all older girls and women have periods, and all older boys and men know about them too.

I'm worried about starting my periods?

Starting your periods is a big event for every girl and is something you will always remember. It shows that you are really growing up. However, starting your periods can also make you feel worried and perhaps a bit scared. So, if you still have questions after reading this section, ask someone, perhaps your mom, an older sister (if you have one), a friend, or a female teacher. She will remember when she first started her periods and will be happy to give you support and advice.

I'm getting white stuff in my underwear?
Am I starting my periods?

The white stuff (called discharge) is part of the way the vagina cleans itself. You'll begin to get it about a year before you start your periods. It is perfectly normal, so don't be embarrassed about it. When you start your periods you will find this discharge changes through your menstrual cycle (see page 56). A few days before your period it may become thicker and stretchy like raw egg white. The discharge may occasionally feel a bit wet and uncomfortable, but it doesn't smell. If you get smelly discharge or are sore and itchy around your vagina, you will need to see a doctor.

How will I know when I am going to start my periods?

Your periods could start at any time from when you are 8 or 9 to when you're 15 or even older, although most girls start at about 12 years old. These are the signs to look out for which tell you that your periods are going to start soon:

- It is about two years since your breasts began to grow.
- It is about a year since you began to notice white or yellowish stains in your underwear (see left).
- You have got pubic hair and hair under your arms.
- You have suddenly grown much taller.

Unfortunately, none of these things will tell you the exact day your periods will start. They are just a way of knowing that you should be prepared.

How much blood comes out when I have a period?

Periods may sound scary, but you only lose a little bit of blood. The first time you have a period, you will probably just notice a reddish-brown stain in your underwear or on your sheets when you wake up in the morning. In total, you will only lose about 3–5 tablespoons of blood during each period and a period can last from 3 to 8 days, so there's not much each day. At the beginning of your period you will usually bleed more than at the end.

How often will I get a period?

When you first begin your periods your
body is not good at getting the timing
right and you won't know when the
next one will arrive. After a year or
more your periods will begin to settle
into a pattern, with about 28 days
between the first day of one period
and the start of the next. Some girls have
longer cycles than this and some girls shorter.

Note down when you have your
period in a diary, on a calendar, or
using an app on your phone.
After a while you will begin
to notice a pattern called a
menstrual cycle.

Does it hurt to have a period?

Some girls get cramps low down in their tummy and backache.
Holding a hot-water bottle against your tummy or having a warm
bath can make you feel better. Although you may not feel like doing
sport or exercise, it can help. If the pain gets bad, ask a parent or the
school nurse if they can give you a tablet to ease it. If your periods
are very painful and nothing helps to ease the pain, see a doctor.

Do periods make you grumpy?

Remember those chemical messengers called hormones? Hormones
tell your body how to keep changing through your menstrual cycle,
which is the time from one period to the next. These hormones are in

your blood and so they go everywhere and can affect you in all sorts of ways. Just before your period, they may make you feel grumpy or tearful. These hormones can also make your breasts a bit tender, your tummy can feel bloated, and you might get a few pimples (spots). All this is annoying, but normal. It is known as PMS or premenstrual syndrome.

I have started my periods and none of my friends has. Why has it happened to me?

It can be lonely if you start your periods before all your friends because there is no one to share what is happening, but it is perfectly normal. Some girls begin their periods at 8 or 9, others at 15 or even older. Get a parent to talk to your teacher so they know what is happening and can help you with the practicalities, such as making sure there is a sanitary disposal can (bin) in the toilet for your used sanitary napkins (pads), helping you have somewhere private to change for PE, or understanding if you can't go swimming. Before long someone else will have started their periods and then someone else, and soon it will be the girls who haven't started that feel lonely, but they too will start when their bodies are ready.

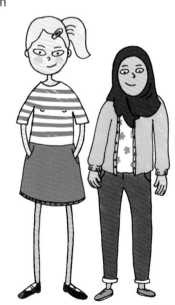

WHAT SHOULD I DO WHEN I HAVE A PERIOD?

Often the biggest worry about starting your periods is coping while still going about your normal daily life. There is no reason to worry, though, as modern sanitary products make it very easy!

What should I do about the blood?

You can either catch the blood in a sanitary napkin (pad), which you stick inside your underwear, or in a tampon that you push inside your vagina. Most girls start with sanitary napkins because these are easier to use. You can buy them from grocery stores. Many sanitary

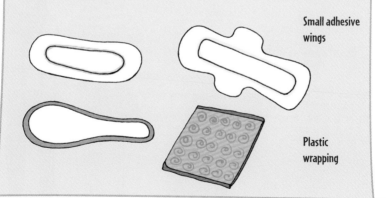

SANITARY NAPKINS (PADS)

Sanitary napkins (pads) come in different shapes and sizes. The type of napkin you use will depend on the heaviness of your period. Some have small adhesive wings at the sides to keep the napkin in place in your underwear.

Many sanitary napkins are individually wrapped in plastic, which makes them easy to carry around.

Small adhesive wings

Plastic wrapping

napkins come individually wrapped in colored wrappers. They are slim and spares slip easily into a schoolbag or pocket. There is an adhesive strip on the back which sticks to your underwear. Some also have adhesive wings which you wrap underneath your underwear.

 ### I've seen sanitary napkins (pads) in stores and they come in different sizes. How do I know which size to get?

Sanitary napkins come in different sizes because your period may be heavier at the beginning and you may need a thicker one. At night, you may also need to use a bigger, thicker napkin, as you won't want to get up and change it every few hours. Look out for sanitary products that are specially designed for young girls and teenagers too.

 ### How often do I need to change my sanitary napkin (pad) and what should I do with the used one?

You will need to change your sanitary napkin about every four hours, and maybe more often at the start of a period. Take off the old napkin, roll it up, put on a new one, and wrap the used one in the wrapper from the new one or in some toilet paper. Some schools and public toilets provide bags for used napkins. Then put the used napkin in the trash. School and public bathrooms usually have sanitary disposal cans (bins); at home, you can put it in the trash can. Never flush sanitary napkins down a toilet because they will block it and that can be embarrassing. Some tampon leaflets state that the tampons are flushable, but they can still block the toilet.

What are tampons?

Tampons are made of a soft absorbent material. They are small and cylinder-shaped to fit inside your vagina. Some are pushed in with your finger, but others have a plunger for pushing them in. If you put tampons in properly, you can't see or feel them, but you may need to practice inserting them. You should change your tampon every few hours, as there is a small risk you can become ill if you leave it in too long. You remove the tampon by pulling on the attached string. Some religions don't allow girls to use tampons.

Tampons fit inside your vagina and soak up the blood. Some have a special applicator, or plunger, for pushing in the tampon. You pull on the string that runs through the tampon to remove it.

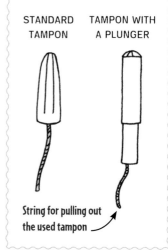

STANDARD TAMPON   TAMPON WITH A PLUNGER

String for pulling out the used tampon

 ## What happens if my period starts at school?

Ask a parent to prepare an emergency pack that you can keep in your bag if you think your periods are about to start. Include some spare underwear and one or two sanitary napkins (pads). If a period starts, and you don't have any sanitary napkins, don't panic. Put some toilet paper in your underwear and go to see the school nurse or a female teacher. Don't be embarrassed. They started their periods once and know just what it feels like.

Will anyone know when I have a period?

No, unless you tell them. Modern sanitary napkins (pads) are slim and invisible when they're in your underwear. Some girls worry about being smelly when on a period, but you won't be smelly if you bath or shower each day and change your napkin or tampon every few hours.

Can I do sport when I have a period?

Yes, you can do everything you normally do. Top athletes do sport when they have a period, and so can you. The only thing you can't do is swim, unless you use a tampon or one of the new types of period-proof swimwear.

BOYS: WHAT HAVE PERIODS GOT TO DO WITH ME?
Boys, you need to know about periods as they can affect your mom, sisters, friends, and other women you know. For example, when a girl has a period she may not want to go swimming; she might get stomach cramps which stop her wanting to go out; she may need a public bathroom, so she can change her sanitary napkin (pad); and she may need a bag with spare napkins. Also, just before a period, she might get a bit moody and bad-tempered. If you know why, you can be more understanding and not ask embarrassing questions.

WHY DO GIRLS SHAVE?

Some girls shave under their arms and/or their legs because they're self-conscious about body hair, but whether you shave is entirely up to you.

 ### Should I shave under my arms?

Most women shave under their arms (or use another method like depilatory cream). It is a small area, so it is easy to do if you want to.

 ### I've got very hairy legs. What can I do about it?

If you decide to shave your legs, then wet shaving or using a depilatory cream are probably the best methods for your age group.

⭐ Shaving is easy, but the hair is prickly when it grows back, and can appear darker and thicker because the ends are blunt. You can also nick yourself and may get in-growing hairs, which can cause pimples (spots).

⭐ Depilatory cream works well, especially for fine hair. You spread it on, leave it for a few minutes to dissolve the hair, then wash it away. The hair is slower to regrow than after shaving. But some people hate the smell and find it messy to use. Some people are also allergic to it.

 ### What should I do about dark hair on my face?

It is best not to shave or pluck this because it may look darker and stronger when it grows back. Instead, try a bleaching cream to lighten the hairs so that they don't show.

TOP TIPS FOR SHAVING

★ Use a sharp razor designed for women (not one of your dad's). You are less likely to cut yourself with a sharp razor because it will glide easily over the skin. Change the razor regularly before it gets blunt.

★ Never share someone else's razor because this can lead to infections.

★ Give yourself plenty of time to shave, as rushing can result in painful nicks.

★ Shave your legs in the shower or bathtub when the hair is warm and soft. Use a shaving gel or lotion on your skin so that the razor glides over it smoothly. If you shave in the shower, put your foot up on a stool, so you can see what you are doing.

★ Shave upward from the ankle, shaving against the hair growth. Pull the skin tight with the other hand as you shave.

★ Use a mirror if you are shaving under your arm, so you can clearly see what you are doing.

★ Only use moisturizing cream on your legs a few hours after you have shaved them. It may sting and irritate your skin if you use one straightaway.

★ Don't use deodorant or antiperspirant straight after shaving under your arms because it will sting.

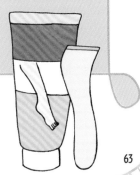

Some girls like to use a depilatory cream to remove hair from their legs or under their arms. It dissolves the hairs and is easy to wash away.

CHAPTER 4

BOYS AND PUBERTY

Boys, this is a chapter just for you (although girls may want
to read it too, so they know what's going on with their
brothers and their male friends and classmates). It deals
mainly with your penis and testicles, as they will probably
become a big focus of your life when you reach puberty. It
tells you how they change, how they behave, and what is
normal. There's also a section on shaving and the
embarrassing moments when your voice sounds like it
is out of your control.

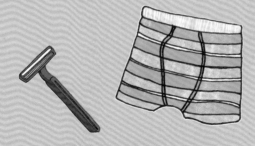

MY PENIS AND ME

During puberty you may begin to think about your penis a lot. Your penis changes shape and size, and also begins to behave in strange ways which can be surprising and embarrassing.

 I keep getting erections and it is really embarrassing. What should I do about them?

Once you begin puberty and your genitals start to develop, your penis gets a mind of its own and you start having erections (see page 25) at embarrassing times, for no reason. This is perfectly normal. If you do have an erection, try to think of something boring, such as practicing your times tables, trying to remember all the soccer scores from the previous weeks' matches, or planning your homework, and your penis will go down. Also find ways of covering up the erection. For example, if it happens on the beach, hold a towel casually in front of you. If you're at school, try untucking your shirt or, if you're sitting down, pick up your school bag, put it on your lap, and pretend to look for something inside.

 What is a wet dream?

At some point during puberty, after your testicles start producing sperm, you might wake up one morning and find that your pajamas or sheet are wet and sticky. Don't worry, you haven't wet the bed! You have had a wet dream. Semen containing sperm (see page 130) has been released from your penis. This is called ejaculation. Some boys have a lot of wet dreams, while some have none at all. Both are completely normal.

What should I do if I have a wet dream?

If you have a wet dream, simply change your sleepwear and wash it with your other clothes. The amount of wetness is quite small and it's not at all like wetting the bed. It's a good idea to start changing your clothes frequently anyway because puberty can make you a bit smelly, so a little extra laundry after a wet dream won't be too much trouble.

My friend says he's circumcised. What does this mean?

The head of the penis is covered by loose skin called the foreskin, which can be pulled back. The foreskin pulls back automatically when you have an erection and should be pulled back when you are washing your penis (see page 33). Circumcision is the name of an operation in which this skin is cut off when you are a baby. Many baby boys in the US are circumcised because their parents prefer it. Some religions say that baby boys must be circumcised and, very occasionally, it is done for medical reasons. If you have a foreskin and your friend hasn't, your penises will look a bit different.

Should I be worried that my penis is much smaller than my friend's?

You see your friends' faces all the time, so you don't worry about comparing the sticking-out bits like your nose or ears. Penises are kept covered, so they are more of a mystery. They are also very important to boys, so when you pee together or shower together after sport, you try to compare them. If you have started puberty, your penis will have begun to grow longer. If you are well into puberty, your penis will be wider as well. If you haven't started puberty yet, your penis will be much smaller than the boys who have started. Also the size of your penis when it is relaxed is not related to how big it is when it is erect. Most adult men have penises that are about the same size when they are erect.

At your age, the differences in your penises will depend on how far into puberty you and your friends are. Penises are different shapes and sizes, just like noses and ears, but many boys think bigger is better. That isn't true.

A few men have smaller or larger penises, but the size of your penis will make no difference later in life when you have a sexual relationship. Just as you can't change how tall you are or the size of your feet, so you can't change the size of your penis, and you should accept it as part of who you are.

It feels nice to rub my penis. Is it wrong to do this?

Since you were a little boy you have probably comforted yourself by holding your penis and discovered how nice it feels, but your parents will have told you not to touch your penis in public. Rubbing your penis is called masturbation, and it is okay to do it in private. All boys do it. When your testicles have started to produce sperm, you'll find that when you masturbate it starts feeling nicer and nicer. Then suddenly you ejaculate (semen comes out of your penis). This will be a surprise the first time it happens. It is called "coming" or having an orgasm, and is what happens when you have sex. Both boys and girls masturbate, boys by rubbing their penises, girls by rubbing their clitorises (see page 53).

As you go through puberty, your penis will get longer and thicker. Don't worry about the size of your penis or compare it with your friends' because you will all develop at different times.

MY TESTICLES AND ME

Testicles are strange organs that dangle outside the body. When it's hot, they hang low; when it's cold, they shrink. If you accidentally crush them, it hurts till you cry. What are they all about?

Why does it hurt so much if you get hit in the testicles?

All boys know how much it hurts if you get hit or kicked in the testicles. The pain doesn't stay in the balls, but travels up into the body; it can make you cry and even make you sick. Testicles are strange organs. Body temperature is too high for sperm and kills them, so testicles have to dangle outside the body to keep them at a lower temperature. This means that, unlike all your other organs, they have no bones to protect them. They are also full of nerves. This makes your testicles feel nice when they are touched, but hurt badly when they are banged or squashed.

Should I wear protection for my testicles when I do sport?

In the past, boys used to wear jock straps or athletic supports for their genitals. These days firm, elasticated sportswear does the job instead. For some sports (e.g. baseball or cricket) boys wear a plastic cup (called an abdo guard or box) over their penis and testicles, which is held in place by their underwear.

One of my testicles looks bigger than the other and hangs down lower. Is this normal?

Testicles grow to be about 2–3 inches (5–7.5cm) long and 1 inch (2.5cm) wide. Most men have one testicle that is bigger than the other, and it is usually the right testicle that is bigger than the left. Also one testicle, usually the left, hangs lower than the one on the right. This is normal.

A few things can go wrong with testicles, and some of them are quite serious, so if one of your testicles (or both) becomes swollen or painful you should tell your parents straightaway and see a doctor quickly.

Why do my testicles seem to shrink sometimes?

The body is very clever because it makes sure that the sperm in testicles are kept at the correct temperature. If the testicles get cold, such as when you swim in cold water, the scrotum is automatically pulled up closer to the warmth of the body and the scrotum looks smaller and more wrinkly. When it is very hot the scrotum dangles down lower into the breeze!

SHAVING, MAN BREASTS, AND SQUEAKY VOICES

Stubble, six packs, and deep voices, that's how lots of men look in movies, but in puberty things can seem to go wrong for a while. Don't worry, this is only a stage which you will soon get through.

 ## I'm beginning to get a mustache. Should I start shaving?

When you first shave is up to you. The first hair that you will get on your upper lip and chin is often known as peach fuzz. This is soft, like the hair on the skin of a peach, but makes a noticeable shadow, especially if you have very dark hair. This hair will gradually become thicker and stronger. Most boys don't shave until they are well into their teens, but if having this hair begins to embarrass you, it may be time to start shaving. Ask a parent or older brother to help you buy a new razor and some shaving gel or an electric shaver, and teach you how to shave well.

 ## Help! I think I'm growing man breasts!

One effect of hormones in puberty is that lots of boys get a slight growth like the beginning of breasts under their nipples. These will remain as small bumps and won't get bigger like breasts in girls. The bumps will disappear as you get older, usually within one or two years. They are probably barely noticeable to other people but, if you feel self-conscious about them, wear loose T-shirts.

People say my voice is breaking. What does that mean?

You have an organ called a larynx (voice box) in your throat. Inside are two stretched muscles called vocal cords, which are a bit like elastic bands. When you speak, air from your lungs rushes over the vocal cords and makes them vibrate. Try plucking a short, thin elastic band when it is stretched tight and you'll find it makes a high-pitched twang. A thicker, longer one makes a much lower note. In puberty, your vocal chords grow longer and thicker, so you begin to speak with a much deeper voice. At the same time, the bones in your face grow and create spaces inside your head. These make the sound louder in the same way that the hollow body of a guitar does.

WHAT IS AN ADAM'S APPLE?
When you look in the mirror, you may notice a lump in your throat that moves up and down when you talk. This is called your Adam's apple. It is actually your bigger larynx, which grew as your voice broke. As the larynx grows, it changes position slightly so that it sticks out of the front of your neck.

Unfortunately, the change from having a high voice to a low one doesn't always happen smoothly. For a few months your voice may be deep one moment and go squeaky the next. If people point it out, just laugh it off and be reassured that it will soon settle down.

CHAPTER 5

LOOKING AFTER YOUR MIND

It's not only your body that changes in puberty. Your brain does too and these changes, together with the effects of all the hormones pumping around in your blood, can make life seem very confusing. This chapter deals with the ups and downs of life at your age, from arguing with parents to feeling sad or bad about yourself, and gives you ways to help yourself when things get difficult.

WHY DO TEENAGERS ACT DIFFERENTLY?

Like your body, your brain changes dramatically in puberty. It grows and wires itself up with millions of new "neural pathways" (connections), which will gradually get you thinking and behaving like an adult. It is also affected by all those hormones racing through your bloodstream, which can result in lots of up-and-down emotions.

Here's a list of things that teenagers might sometimes say or think. Which ones do you agree with?

⭐ I hate my nose/chin/breasts/hair/eyebrows...

⭐ All my friends are better-looking than me.

⭐ I wish I could be like xxxxxxx.

⭐ I'm proud of what I've achieved at school/in sport/in music...

⭐ I hate the way my parents are always on at me...

⭐ I love the way that I'm allowed more independence now.

⭐ I wish I was allowed more independence.

⭐ I hate that my friends have more independence than me.

⭐ I want to do things with my friends, not my family.

⭐ My family are great and we have fun together.

⭐ I'm worried that my parents will get ill.

⭐ I get angry when my parents don't respect my privacy.

⭐ I'm ashamed of things I've done and said just to impress my friends.

⭐ I often feel lonely.

⭐ I fancy someone, but I don't know what to say to them.

⭐ If I speak out in class, I worry people will laugh at me.

⭐ I hate getting up in the mornings.

⭐ Sometimes I'm really happy and the next moment I feel depressed.

⭐ Nobody likes me and I think they all talk about me behind my back.

⭐ I have a real laugh with my friends.

You and your friends could probably add more. Just knowing other people feel the same can help you deal with confusing emotions, but in this chapter we suggest ways of coping when things get hard.

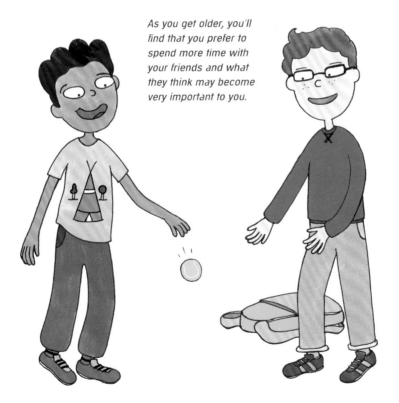

As you get older, you'll find that you prefer to spend more time with your friends and what they think may become very important to you.

What can I do if I'm always arguing with my parents?

Think of your brain as having two parts. The emotional part says, "Go on/have fun/that'll be cool/ don't be a wimp/I really want that." The thinking part says, "Whoa/that could be dangerous/that's bad/that could hurt someone's feelings/ that's really expensive." It's a battle and, at your age, the emotional part is more likely to win. You end up acting without thinking,

Most young people argue with their parents about things like phones and screen time, privacy (both on- and off-line), tidying their bedroom, doing homework, bed times, what to wear, and the stuff that everyone else has and you want.

taking risks, and saying things that get you into trouble and which will upset your parents. Your brain is also saying, "Come on, it's time to be more independent, time to spend more time with your friends, try out new things, and become a different person from the little kid you used to be." This is hard for your parents and can lead to arguments.

When you are angry, try breathing deeply and counting to ten before you speak, and get that thinking part of your brain working. A discussion is always better than an argument. Try to remember that, even though the decisions your parents make may seem unfair and too strict, you still need them because they are the ones who care for you and believe in you. The rules they set are there to keep you safe and help you grow up into a successful adult.

Young people who talk with their parents are usually happier than those who don't, but this can be difficult when your parents are very busy. They may not realize that they are not always available to talk to you, so you may have to ask them to give you some time and point it out to them if they are on their phones a lot!

People keep telling me to try things, but I can't be bothered. Why should I?

Your brain is doing amazing things. It's growing and becoming more powerful by wiring itself up with millions of new connections, which means sports, musical instruments, and languages are easier to learn now than when you are older. Your thinking power is also expanding, so puberty is a great time to try new things. If you are worried about missing out on time with your friends, try to get them to come with you. Being successful at something different will boost your confidence and help you make new friends (see page 94). Don't worry that you won't be good at it; you won't know until you try. But, remember, nobody can make you do anything you don't want to.

Puberty gives your brain a boost, so use your new thinking powers to get involved in new projects, debate big issues (perhaps join the debating club at school), and save the world!

WILL I GET INTO BAD MOODS?

Watch any drama about young people and you will see plenty of sighing, scowling, and door slamming. Puberty is a time when bad moods can make life difficult, but there is always a way through them.

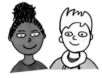 **One moment I'm happy, the next I want to cry. Is there something wrong with me?**

No! That's just your hormones affecting your brain. Hormones make you more self-conscious, so you may think everyone is looking at you and judging you, which makes you feel embarrassed. Changes in your brain also make you see yourself and others in a different way. You might feel no one understands you. You might fall out with friends. You might feel you have a problem that you can't solve.

On the other hand, when something goes well, you can feel fantastic. Puberty is a confusing time and it's similar for everyone. However confident your friends may seem, they'll be having similar worries and mood swings as you. When things feel bad, find someone that you trust to talk to. Try your mom, dad, grandma, grandad, carer, teacher, sports coach, older sibling, or a friend. Sometimes strong emotions can feel overwhelming and hard to cope with. You can do other things to help you cope, such as slowing down your breathing (see page 86), writing worries down, or doing a calming activity like drawing or coloring. Find what works for you.

Writing your thoughts down in a notebook can often help if you are upset or annoyed about something.

I feel sad all the time. What should I do?

Things happen that make us feel sad. For example, it can be very difficult and sad if somebody close to you dies or if your parents get divorced. Lots of other things will make you sad, and you can't always be happy, but you shouldn't feel sad or low all the time. Even if you can't pinpoint what is making you sad, it is best to talk about how you are feeling, either with somebody you know and trust (see opposite) or with an expert (see page 83). If you feel like hurting yourself, it is even more important to talk to someone and ask for help. There is always help available and you won't feel like this forever.

What should I do if I feel aggressive?

You need to find a way to deal with it. Give yourself time. Walk away from whoever has made you angry. Shut yourself in your room and punch a pillow or listen to music while you calm down. Slow your breathing (see page 86). Then try to talk calmly about what made you angry. Remember: anger is an important emotion and there are lots of reasons to be angry. It is better to let anger out than to keep it inside where it builds up, but it is never okay to hit out and be aggressive. If you keep feeling aggressive or finding yourself arguing or fighting, think about whether you have been spending a lot of time playing violent computer games. Young people who play these games for hours are more likely to be aggressive in real life, so it might be worth cutting down on these and doing something active instead. Physical activities can use up energy and aggression.

WHY DO I FEEL WORRIED ALL THE TIME?

Everyone worries. Events such as changing schools, moving house, parents arguing, bust-ups with mates, bullying, problems with schoolwork, and illness are always worrying. At puberty you may begin to worry about different things, too. What your friends think of you and how you compare to other people become much more important.

How can I deal with my worries?

Not all worries are the same. Some are about taking risks: starting a new school, raising your hand in class, trying out for a school play, or joining a new sports club can all make you worry, but get through the challenge and you will feel great! Overcoming these worries makes you feel more confident and better about yourself. Some worries can be sorted with help from other people. Here are some things you can try to help you deal with various worries:

- ⭐ If you are having problems with your schoolwork, talk to your parents or a teacher (see Box, opposite).
- ⭐ If you've fallen out with a friend, make the first move to work things out. Say sorry and discuss together how you can move on.
- ⭐ If you are frightened of getting into trouble for something you've done wrong, be brave, admit to it, and find out how to put things right.

What should I do if I feel I can't solve my worries?

Some worries can't be solved easily. Parents do get divorced. Not all parents are kind to their children. People do get ill and die. There are experts who can help if you are worried about issues like these (see

Box, below). The main thing to remember is *all worries need to be talked about*. Sharing them can cut them down in size, make you feel less alone, and often throw up solutions. Writing worries down can do the same for some people. Remember, facing up to and getting through your worries will make you stronger and more grown-up.

TALKING ABOUT YOUR WORRIES

People may suggest that you should talk to an adult about your worries, but you might not know where to start. It's normal to feel nervous about talking to someone you don't know well about a difficult subject. Whether you're talking to a teacher, doctor, or someone on a helpline, remember they have had these kinds of conversations with many young people before and will want to help you to feel less nervous. If you don't know what to say, they will ask you questions. Try to be as honest as possible, and tell them the problem and what your worries are. Write it down if that is easier than saying it. (See page 140 for a list of organizations you can contact if you need help.)

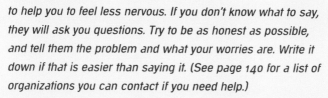

STRESS AND ANXIETY

You hear the word stress a lot. Everyone can be stressed, but too much stress is bad for you and you need to learn how to deal with it.

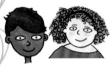

What is stress?

Stress is when worrying thoughts keep coming back and start affecting your whole life. Sometimes, people who are stressed:

⭐ Can't relax.

⭐ Find it hard to concentrate.

⭐ Can't get to sleep.

⭐ Get bad-tempered or cry a lot.

⭐ Go off their food or eat all the time.

⭐ Get headaches or tummy aches.

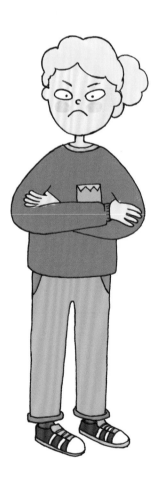

If you think you're stressed, then you need to do two things. Talk through your worries (see page 83) and learn to relax (see Box, opposite). Relaxing properly is not easy and it helps to practice every day.

When you are going through puberty, you may find that you become more stressed and anxious. People who feel stressed can also be grumpy and irritable.

DIFFERENT WAYS TO RELAX

You can relax by doing things you enjoy, especially active things. Have a go at these and see if they help you feel more relaxed:

* ⭐ *Bounce on your trampoline.*
* ⭐ *Stroke your cat.*
* ⭐ *Take your dog for a walk.*
* ⭐ *Put on some loud music and dance.*
* ⭐ *Watch a funny cat on YouTube and laugh out loud.*
* ⭐ *Kick a ball around.*
* ⭐ *Learn to meditate.*
* ⭐ *Slow down your breathing (see page 86).*
* ⭐ *Get plenty of sleep (see page 44).*
* ⭐ *Think about times when you've been really happy.*

What is a panic attack?

To panic is natural. It is the body's way of getting us out of danger by making our hearts beat faster and our breathing get quicker, so that we can run away to safety. That was fine in the past when the danger was a wild animal, for example, but is not so great when you are panicking about a test you have coming up or going into school after you have been bullied. A panic attack isn't just worry. It affects your whole body, as well as your heart and breathing. This is what can happen:

- ⭐ Your mouth goes dry.
- ⭐ You feel breathless, sick, or dizzy.
- ⭐ You need to pee.
- ⭐ You can't think clearly or concentrate.
- ⭐ You may feel so bad that you think you're really ill and are going to faint or have a heart attack. This won't happen.

Your body is telling you to run, but that's not going to help you pass that test or face going into school, so you need to work through the panic. To do this, you must slow down your breathing to get it back to normal and distract you from the worry (see Box, below).

HOW TO SLOW DOWN YOUR BREATHING
- ⭐ Close your eyes and breathe out.
- ⭐ Breathe in as you count slowly to five.
- ⭐ Hold your breath for a count of two.
- ⭐ Breathe out for another slow count of five.
- ⭐ Repeat this five or six times.

BOOSTING YOUR SELF-ESTEEM

Self-esteem is how you feel about yourself. Some people have high self-esteem, while others struggle and feel bad about themselves. Try to believe in yourself because this can help give you a positive attitude to life.

 ## What is self-esteem and why does it matter?

Young people who have high self-esteem are confident and happy because they are realistic, but positive, about themselves and what they can achieve. Young people with low self-esteem are low in confidence and think they are useless. No one should feel that way. The best boost for your self-esteem is when other people say nice things about you, but you can also do a lot to help yourself. Try these things to boost your self-esteem:

⭐ Try not to compare your looks to celebrities or the best-looking people in your class. Be attractive in your own way. Present yourself well (see pages 28–31 for advice on keeping yourself clean), look people in the eye, and smile. Act as if you are confident in who you are, even when you are scared inside.

⭐ Think about what you are good at. It may be something in school like history or sport, or it may be something completely different like inventing games or looking after younger children. Whatever it is, be proud of your successes and keep building on them.

⭐ Don't dwell on your failures. Accept them and move on in small steps to get better at the things you're not so good at. Be proud of every step you take. Try new activities, which may turn out to be things you're really good at.

⭐ Be a good friend and be proud of it. Good friends listen, support, keep secrets, and are loyal and kind. They don't join in cruel gossip or bullying behavior.

⭐ Finish every day by listing three things that went well or made you happy.

CHAPTER 6

WE ARE ALL DIFFERENT

This chapter covers loads of different subjects because,
as the title says, we are all different and worry about
different things. At your age you will probably spend a lot
of time thinking about yourself and what other people
think of you. You may worry about everything, from your
appearance, to friends, to boyfriends or girlfriends, and
what it means to be a boy or a girl. This chapter deals
with some of those worries.

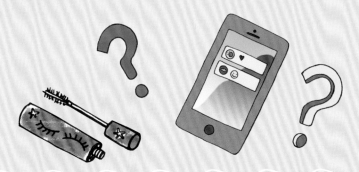

IT'S SO... EMBARRASSING: YOUR CHANGING BODY

Bodies come in all shapes and sizes, and that is even more true when some people have started puberty and others haven't. At the same time, you begin to feel more self-conscious and you wonder why you can't look like the people you see on YouTube or in movies. It's not always easy to be happy with your changing body.

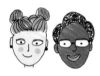

My friend is really skinny and I feel ginormous beside her. What can I do?

Remember that the age at which puberty begins is different for different people (see page 13). If you've started puberty before your friend, you are going to grow faster. Boys will get taller and broader, and they are usually proud to be like this. Girls will get taller and their breasts, hips, thighs, and bum will also get curvier. Some girls find these changes worrying, but you need to be proud too. It is really important that you eat healthily and don't try to diet to stop your body changing. Whatever you are like now, you won't know how

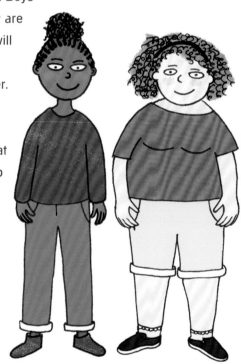

you will end up as an adult. Your final shape will depend partly on your genes (see page 133) and partly on your weight. You can't change your genes, but if you are feeling "ginormous" because you're overweight (and a doctor or nurse has told you that you need to lose weight), then you should get help and advice on eating a healthy diet (see page 36) and getting more exercise (see page 40).

I hate my nose. I'd do anything to change it!

When you're going through puberty you become very self-conscious. You begin to spend a lot of time in front of the mirror or taking selfies, and the more you look at yourself, the more you find not to like. Don't worry about bits of you!

It's not easy but, remember, the things you don't like about yourself may be the things that make you special and also turn out to be the very things that someone falls in love with.

The people who look really good are the ones who are confident about who they are. It doesn't matter how big your nose is, or your chin or your bum, or if your hair is straight or curly, if you can say, "I like being who I am."

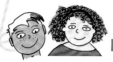

Everyone in my class is taller/shorter than me

In any class there are always some people who are short, some who are tall, and a lot who are in the middle. The shortest and the tallest people often feel self-conscious. Girls often begin puberty and have their growth spurt before boys so, in a class of 11 year olds, a lot of the girls will be taller than the boys, but by age 15 most of the boys will be taller than the girls. Boys who used to be the smallest in their class will reach puberty and suddenly grow and broaden. Girls who used to be the tallest may stop growing, while others keep going. How tall you end up mostly depends on how tall your parents are because it is mostly your genes (see page 133) that decide your height and you can't change those.

Try not to worry about your height. If people tease you, try to answer them in a way that shows you don't care. Find a hero who is short or tall, and you can say, "Xxxxxxx is really short/tall and he/she has done okay!"

Children your age will be different heights, but this is nothing to worry about.

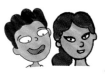 **I'm worried that people will think that I'm ugly if I have to wear braces or glasses?**

Lots of young people are advised by their dentist to wear braces to straighten their adult teeth. If you have to, it will be worth it because the result will be a beautiful smile, and you'll soon get used to wearing them.

If you have to wear glasses, you'll soon get over feeling self-conscious and these days glasses can be cool! You might not have to wear them all the time; it depends on your eyes. You can wear contact lenses, but you must keep them clean. In summer, everyone should wear shades to protect their eyes from the sun.

How will my disability affect going through puberty?

If you have a disability or health condition, you will usually go through puberty in the same way as everyone else. You may have different challenges, but, as this chapter shows, all young people have their own challenges. To understand more about how your disability may affect how you go through puberty, talk with your parents or doctor.

HOW CAN I MAKE PEOPLE LIKE ME?

Life isn't fair. Some people are popular and have loads of friends, while other find it harder to make and keep friends. If you're feeling that you don't have friends, here are ten tips that might help.

1 Remember the rules of friendship you learnt when you were younger: share and take turns, be kind, don't be bossy, don't show off, and don't lash out or get angry if things don't go your way.

2 Be yourself. Stick to your own interests, beliefs, and ideas. You have your own character and you won't be as respected if you always change to fit in with other people.

3 Accept that the very popular in-crowd may not be right for you and there are better people to be friends with.

4 Be friendly to everyone, smile, and chat. Excluding other "uncool" people won't make you cool.

5 Try new activities, and find and share new music, games, and videos. This will give you the chance to make new friends and give you plenty to talk about.

6 Work out conversation openers to use when you meet new people.

7 Be a good listener. If you're not confident about what to say, encourage other people to do the talking.

8 Be funny and make jokes (not unkind ones). Don't be afraid to laugh at yourself and if someone makes a joke about you, try to laugh it off and send one back.

9 Compliment people, and don't put them down. A put-down may get you a quick laugh, but it won't win you friends. Nobody is really confident inside, so a compliment will make them feel good and open to your friendship.

10 Find something you're good at and get even better at it. People will respect you and you may find other people who share your passion.

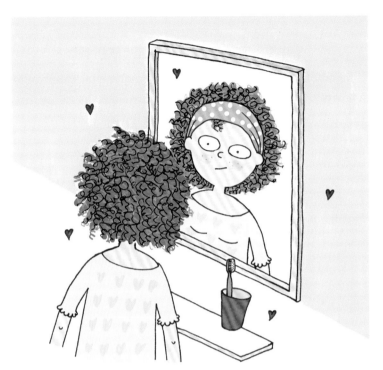

You may find yourself worrying that you're not popular, or if you've fallen out with a friend. Try not to worry too much and remember always to be yourself.

Finally, if you are sad about friendships that go wrong, or people not being nice to you, talk to an adult about it. Adults were your age once and went through the same things as you're going through. They will be able to help.

FRIENDS, GEEKS, AND CLIQUES

In puberty, friends become more and more important to you. What they think often matters much more than what your parents or teachers think. But friendships are not always easy.

Is it good to have a best friend?

Best friends can be great. You feel comfortable with your best friend, share a laugh, have fun together, and chat for hours. Best friends look out for you and you can trust them. Having a best friend can also teach you about arguing and making up, not getting your own way, and understanding someone else, but having just one best friend can be a problem. A group of good friends is probably better. Think about these points:

⭐ You and your best friend can become a clique which excludes others and makes them unhappy.

⭐ Your best friend can become possessive and stop you being friends with and doing things with other people.

⭐ You can spend hours sharing worries with your best friend, but don't talk about how to make things better. You end up making each other more worried.

⭐ If you come to depend on one best friend, you may find it hard to make new friends if the friendship breaks up or your friend moves away.

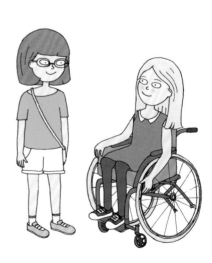

My friend keeps being horrible to me. What should I do?

It can be very hard if your friend
starts being horrible to you,
especially if you don't
understand why. Working out
what to do isn't easy either.
You may feel that if you break
up your friendship you will be
left without a friend, but you also need

Some friends end up being more
like enemies because they put you
down, laugh at you, leave you out,
or do other mean things. This can
really hurt if the person used to be
a good friend and has changed.

to stand up for yourself. Don't just say, "You are being
mean to me," but start with an "I." Try saying, "I don't like the way
you keep putting me down and laughing at me in front of other
people. If you keep doing it, I won't be your friend anymore."

Your "friend" might take this as a chance to end your friendship,
but that might be better than being in a friendship that makes you
unhappy. Alternatively, your friend may realize that he/she needs
your friendship and start being nice to you, especially as you've
shown that you are strong enough to stand up to him/her.

I've been called a geek just because I like science and computers. What should I say?

If you're really interested in your schoolwork (or in computers or
some other subject), and are less interested in hanging out with

friends or doing sport, then you may find that other people call you a geek or a nerd. All name-calling is cruel, but if you have been called names like these, then pause and think things through a bit. Can you feel proud instead of hurt? Remember that:

★ Today, geeks and nerds rule the world through tech companies like Microsoft and Apple.

★ Although it's great to be good at sport, few people make it into top teams.

★ It's fun to hang out with friends, but it could stop you getting good grades at school. Which is more important?

★ Cool people at school, who make fun of nerds and geeks, may find that they are left behind when it comes to life beyond school.

You can tell people all these things when they mock you, but you should also be careful not to spend too much time on your own, especially in front of a screen. Everyone needs to learn to make friends and everyone should spend time being active. You need to find a balance.

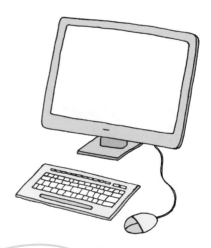

Why are cliques bad?

Most young people
have a group of
friends who they
hang out with at
school or at home.
They are all individuals who do their
own things and, although they may fall out at times and
have arguments, they generally like and support each other.
Cliques are different from these groups. Here is what
can happen in a clique:

If you are part of a clique, you may be very happy, but you might be making others unhappy or you might be letting yourself down by behaving in ways you know are wrong. Think about it!

- People in a clique do everything together. They wear the same fashions and say that they like the same things.

- Often there is a leader in the clique who makes the rules and decides who can and can't belong.

- A clique excludes other people and the people who do belong often worry about saying or doing the wrong thing in case they are excluded too.

- People in cliques often end up buying clothes they can't afford, taking part in bullying, or doing other things they know they shouldn't.

WHAT IS PEER PRESSURE?

When you do something just because your friends (your peers) do it, that's giving in to peer pressure. It will happen more often as you go through puberty and what your friends think of you starts becoming really important. Peer pressure works for three main reasons: you want to fit in; you want to be liked; and you are afraid other people will make fun of you if you don't join in.

  ## Can peer pressure be a good and bad thing?

Sometimes peer pressure can be good for you, encouraging you to try new activities, become more independent, or work harder at a sport or at school. It can make you dress in a different style, find new types of music, play different games, and make new friends. At other times, the pressure is to do risky things, such as shoplifting or bullying, which you know are wrong and could get you into trouble. You may feel pressured into doing things that could harm you, like smoking, drinking alcohol, or taking drugs. These may sound a smart idea, but your rational mind (see page 78) should ask if it is really cool to:

⭐ Run across the road and get hit by a car? ⭐ Shoplift and get a police record?

⭐ Get drunk and vomit? ⭐ Try drugs and end up in hospital?

How can I get out of things I don't want to do?

If you're a boy, you may feel a lot of peer pressure to be strong and brave, and do risky things that could get you hurt. Boys often worry that if they don't join in, they'll be called "gay" or a "wuss." Girls are often pressured by threats of exclusion. To get out of difficult situations, here are some ideas for what you could say or do:

1 Firmly say, "No, that's a stupid idea," and walk away. Show you are strong and confident in your decision.

2 Give a good reason. "I don't want to risk hurting myself because I'm playing in the team tomorrow."

3 Some people can make a joke. Laughter will take the pressure off.

4 Suggest a better activity. That will help your friends get out of doing it too.

5 Give an excuse, such as "I've got to be home at 4 o'clock."

6 Team up with people who think like you, as it will be easier to walk away together.

If, after you've said that you don't want to be involved, people continue to put pressure on you, calling you names or taunting you, repeat what you said before and walk away.

 ## Why do boys and girls behave differently?

Boys and girls often behave differently, partly because of their hormones and partly because of the way adults treat them as they grow up (see page 104). Boys and girls often (but not always) behave differently with friends. Although many girls do active things together, they're also more likely to talk about relationships, share secrets and emotions, and hug each other. Boys are more likely to play competitive games and sports (although many do not); talk about subjects, not relationships; and joke about and wrestle, rather than hug. Some also take more risks and, at your age, get injured more often, but there are no rules for how boys and girls should behave.

WHAT IS GENDER?

Gender is more than being born a boy or a girl. It's about what it means to be a boy or a girl and how the way you are treated may make you behave in certain ways. It can start very early. Many baby girls are dressed in pink and frills, and baby boys in blue. Little girls often dress up in sparkly dresses and play princesses, while little boys dress up as superheroes and save the world. Girls may be told they're pretty, boys that they're strong.

What has gender got to do with me?

Gender stereotypes are ideas that people have about what boys and girls are supposed to like and do. Look at your toys and possessions. If you are a girl, how many of your things are pink? Even active things like bikes are produced in pink for girls and in dark, more "macho" colors for boys. As you get older, all this affects what you choose to do in life. In many ways, it was worse in the past because boys and girl were expected to lead completely different lives:

⭐ Things were especially bad for girls in the past. They were considered less clever than boys and often did not get a proper education (and they still don't in many parts of the world).

⭐ When girls grew up, they were supposed to get married, stay at home, do housework, look after children, and obey their husbands.

⭐ Boys got an education and went out to work, but it wasn't always easy for boys either. They were supposed to be strong and confident all the time and were not allowed to show their emotions.

Luckily, all that is changing. Now, when you grow up, whether you're a girl or a boy, you can work to be anything you want, so don't let anyone stop you!

ACTIVITIES FOR ALL

Playing soccer, skateboarding, drawing, watching Disney movies, making robots, dressing up, acting, singing, caring for pets, playing computer games, looking after younger siblings, playing an instrument, cooking, making models, sewing, reading, climbing trees, martial arts, dancing, styling your hair, looking at fashion magazines, writing stories, doing science experiments.

Can you split these into boys' and girls' activities? Of course not. Boys and girls can enjoy and be equally good at all of them, but some people might say some of these activities are more suitable for boys than girls or the other way round. What people think may stop you doing what you want to do, wearing what you want to wear, or playing the games you want to play. Sometimes it can be hard to go against expectations. People can laugh at you or call you nasty names but be confident in what you are doing and true to yourself.

Do I have to look a certain way if I'm a girl/boy?

Gender stereotypes can affect the way you look. Girls may think they should wear makeup and high heels, boys that they should be cool and tough, but you should find your own style. Don't try to look like people in videos or adverts, as they are dressed, made up, and posed to look perfect. Their images are also often Photoshopped so their skin looks smoother or their muscles bigger. Try not to be obsessed about what you look like. It may take time, some mistakes, and arguments with your parents before you find your own style, but you will discover what makes you feel good and gives you the freedom to do the things you want to do.

Are boys more aggressive than girls or is that a gender stereotype too?

When they are young, boys are often more active than girls, and do lots of running around, wrestling, and throwing things. Some like to play with toy guns and enjoy shooting games. As they get older, more boys than girls enjoy violent computer games and movies, but these are fantasies and boys don't try to hurt people any more than girls do. However, men are often more aggressive than women. You can tell that from the news. For some, it may be because of the messages they were given when they were young; being told that men must be strong, powerful, and not show any emotion. Sometimes their fathers and other men were aggressive to them and they were taught that if someone hits them, they should hit them back. Today, things are changing. Boys are being taught that it is okay to be emotional, that boys don't have to be strong, and that it is always better to talk about what makes them angry than to fight.

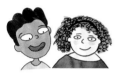

What does transgender mean?

Sometimes children think they have been given the wrong gender. They may have a boy's body but feel inside that they are a girl, so want to be called by a girl's name and wear girl's clothes; or they have a girl's body but feel inside that they are a boy, so they want to have a boy's name and wear boy's clothes. This is different from just enjoying things that are usually enjoyed by children of the opposite gender. Some children feel like they're not a boy or a girl, or that they don't have a gender at all, or that their gender is something different. This is called non-binary.

If you want to talk to somebody about your gender identity, a counselor on one of the helplines (see page 140) is a good place to start. If you feel able to talk to your parents, suggest they read the Mermaids website (see page 140).

It can be very tough for children who have these feelings about their gender. They can get bullied, and even their families may not accept that they feel like this and give them a hard time. If you know someone who is transgender, be kind to them and treat them as just another friend.

BOYFRIENDS, GIRLFRIENDS, AND CRUSHES

When you are younger, boys usually play with boys and girls with girls. As you reach puberty you are much more likely to play or hang out in mixed groups. You begin to tease each other about fancying people and you may have a first boy or girl friend.

When should I have my first boyfriend/girlfriend?

As you get older, you might start fancying someone. You may begin dreaming about holding hands and kissing the person you fancy. Just thinking about them may begin to make you feel tingly and excited inside. Some people may have their first boyfriend or girlfriend. They may spend time alone together, and kissing and cuddling may become part of what they do. However, having a boyfriend or girlfriend can cut you off from your friends and may mean you have less fun. Good friends are more important at your age and they can include someone of the opposite sex who isn't your boyfriend or girlfriend.

Most people don't get their first real boyfriend or girlfriend until later in their teens. The important thing is not to worry if you don't have these feelings and don't fancy someone.

What does it mean to have a crush on someone?

Having a crush is not the same as having a boyfriend or girlfriend. It means there is one person you can't stop thinking about. They seem perfect: beautiful/good-looking, cool, funny, and interested in the things you're interested in. You daydream about them and write their name over and over in your notebook, but when you see them you feel shy and embarrassed and don't know what to say.

Crushes often happen in puberty. Your crush could be the same sex as you or the opposite sex. You could get a crush on a classmate, a girl in an older class, a boy on the bus, a young teacher, the older brother or sister of a friend. It could also be a celebrity. You follow them online, and dream of a time they might notice you. It is all exciting, but confusing.

You may be too shy to talk to your crush. Instead you might tease them, chase them in the playground, write notes, send texts, or buy gifts. You feel desperate to be noticed and just a smile from them can light up your life. Sadly, your crush may not want your attention. They may be older or just not interested. This can really hurt, but you must respect their feelings and not keep hassling them. You may feel like you are dying of a broken heart, but you will get over it!

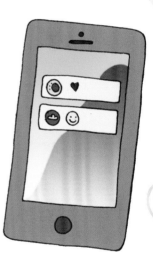

Should I kiss my boyfriend/girlfriend?

Saying that someone is your boyfriend or girlfriend can bring up all sorts of worries. What do you talk about, what do you do together, should you kiss? The idea of kissing makes younger children go "yuk!" Now that you're older, you may want to kiss your boyfriend or girlfriend. If you want to kiss someone, remember to **Ask, Listen, Respec**t, a simple three-step rule:

1 Before you kiss, ask if you may.

2 If he/she says no, listen and respect that decision.

3 Respect means not trying to change his/her mind or ignoring what he/she has said.

Remember: No one should ever be forced to do something they don't want to do. If someone wants to kiss you and you don't want to kiss them, say NO firmly and give your reasons. Just say something like, "I like you, but I'm not ready for kissing yet." (See also page 127.)

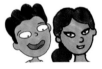 ## What is sexting?

Sexting is sending messages or photos about sex and naked bodies. Sometimes young people sext because other people put pressure on them to send pictures of themselves naked. This is wrong and you should never give into pressure like this, or put pressure on others to send you pictures (see kissing, above). Sexting can start as just a bit of fun. You strip off and try a sexy pose and someone takes a photo. You decide to send it to a girl/boy you like. He/she thinks it's hilarious and shares it with a friend who shares it with someone else and, before you know it, everyone in your school has seen it and is laughing at you. On the internet, there is no delete button. That photo is out there forever. Sexting is very risky. Making or sharing a sexy picture of someone under 18 can be against the law. If somebody has shared a sexual picture of you that you didn't want shared, the police can help you. For more on online safety, see page 124.

What does it mean to be gay and how do I know if I am?

Gay means that you are attracted to people of the same sex rather than the opposite sex, so men are attracted to men and women to women. Bisexual (bi) means you're attracted to both men and women. When you have a crush on someone (see page 106), it is often someone of the same sex because the person is someone you admire and want to be like. This does not mean that you are gay. It means you are trying out different relationships and discovering things about yourself.

It's okay to take some time to figure out who you might be attracted to, and you don't have to define yourself as gay or straight. Just be who you are, and be attracted to whoever you feel attracted to!

Being gay is not something you make a choice about, but something you begin to understand about yourself as you grow up. Some people know they are gay when they are children. Others don't realize it until much later. It is nothing to be ashamed of. Sadly, though, if people think you are gay (whether you are or not), you may get teased and bullied. Saying, "You are so gay" is a way of putting someone down and hurting their feelings. If you think you might be gay or bisexual, you may find it helps to talk to someone (see the helplines n page 140).

CHAPTER 7

STAYING SAFE

Growing up is not just about changes to your body and how you think. It is about becoming independent. This chapter is all about staying safe as you are gradually allowed more freedom. It includes dealing with bullying and cyberbullying, as well as some of the horrible things that can happen to you on- and off-line. It may make freedom sound a bit scary, but if you are prepared, you are much less likely to find yourself in trouble, so be sure to read this chapter.

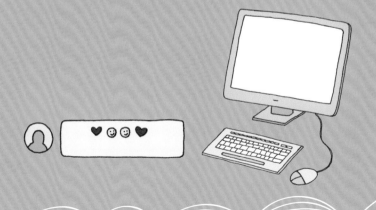

NEW FREEDOMS AND RESPONSIBILITIES

Since you were a baby your parents, carers, and teachers have always taken care of you. Now they may be worried about letting you go into the big, wide world on your own.

 I want more freedom, but my parents are really strict.

More freedom will come to you step by step, but you'll need to "negotiate" (discuss sensibly) each step, and prove to your parents that you can be trustworthy and responsible. Here are 10 freedoms you will need to negotiate, but bear in mind that most young people don't get much freedom before they are 11 years old:

1 **Sleepovers, camps, and residential school trips:** These can be scary if you have never stayed away from home, but they will build your confidence and also your parents' confidence in you.

2 **Playing out:** Is there a place in your street outside your own backyard (garden) where you can ride a bike/skateboard/kick a ball with friends?

3 **Cooking and using knives and other tools:** You might burn or cut yourself, but it's important to develop the skills to look after yourself. Groups like the Scouts (in the UK and US) and Girl Guides (in the UK) are great for learning these skills.

4 **Privacy:** You may want to be able to lock the bathroom door, chat with friends without your parents listening, and have a life at school that they don't know about.

5 **On vacation:** Campsites, vacation complexes, and vacation houses away from the city are often safe places to enjoy new freedoms.

6 **Being home alone:** When you don't want to be dragged out, can you be left home alone for a short time?

7 **Getting a phone:** This is a tough one (see page 116).

8 **Walking or cycling to school or the local store:** If it's only a short walk or a safe cycle to school or a store, can you go alone or call for a friend and go together?

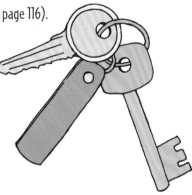

9 **Shopping in the mall/seeing a movie/ going to a sports club:** Can you go with friends without an adult?

10 **Taking public transport:** Can you use this to get to school or to meet friends farther away?

RULES FOR BEING HOME ALONE

You might feel nervous when you are first left at home on your own but there is no need if you are sensible. Now is not the time to start cooking or climbing ladders! Do your homework, read, or watch TV and follow these rules.

1 Keep doors locked and don't open the door to anyone.

2 Only answer phone calls from family.

3 Don't tell anyone that you are home alone.

4 Stay inside and don't ask anyone over.

5 Know who to call in an emergency.

6 Keep in touch with your parents.

How can I get my parents to trust me?

If your parents trust you and are confident that you know what to do if things go wrong, they are more likely to allow you to be independent. Here are some ways to show that you're trustworthy:

⭐ Talk to your parents. Tell them about your friends and what you are doing.

⭐ Show that you can look after your possessions. If you are always losing your sports kit or school bag, will they trust you with a phone or door keys?

⭐ Show that you are responsible. Do your chores and homework without being nagged.

⭐ Keep to rules. Don't try to get round the security they have set up on your computer. Stick to the amount of screen time they allow.

⭐ Ask your friends round to your house and let your parents meet them. If they like and trust your friends, they will trust you more.

⭐ Get your parents together with your friends' parents. If several sets of parents can agree rules about what you and your friends can do, they will be less worried.

⭐ Ask your parents to watch you while you prove you can do things such as crossing the road safely, catching a bus, or riding your bike on the road.

⭐ If you are left home alone, show that you know the rules and follow them (see Box, on page 113).

⭐ If you are allowed out with friends, show that you understand there are dangers, which include people who pretend to be friendly but are not (see page 127). Show that you know the rules and follow them (see Box, opposite).

10 RULES FOR BEING OUT WITH FRIENDS

1 Stay with your friends at all times and never go off with anyone else, even if you know them.

2 Tell your parents where you are and answer your phone if they call or message you. Agree a code word/sentence with your parents to text or phone if you are worried and need somebody to pick you up.

3 Know how to cross roads safely. Use marked crosswalks (pedestrian crossings) whenever you can and stay off your phone as you cross.

4 Keep valuables out of sight. Don't "flash the cash" or walk and talk. This can make you a target for crime. Be aware of what's going on around you.

5 If someone tries to take your money or phone, don't try to fight back.

6 Learn the phone numbers of two people to call in an emergency, as your phone might get lost or stolen, or the battery might go flat.

7 If a stranger asks for help, or tries to be friendly, don't reply and move quickly to a safe place such as a store. Adults should never ask children for help.

8 If a car stops near you, keep walking fast and move to the back of the sidewalk (pavement) where you can't be grabbed.

9 If anyone tries to grab you, scream very loudly, remembering the three Ls: low, loud, and long. Practice at home.

10 Always be home at the time you have agreed. If you are delayed for any reason, let your parents know.

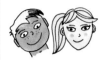

How can I persuade my parents to let me have a phone?

If your parents don't want you to have a phone, it won't be easy. Many adults think phones are bad for young people. Here are some starting points for discussions:

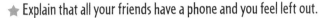

⭐ Explain that all your friends have a phone and you feel left out.

⭐ Talk about how much a phone costs and offer to help pay for your contract by doing chores around the house.

⭐ Prove that you can be trusted to look after a phone properly.

⭐ Promise to stick to any rules your parents make about using the phone (e.g. not using it during mealtimes, at night in bed, or when you're doing homework).

⭐ Talk about safety and promise your parents that they can set your security settings and know your passcode.

If you have a phone, the following rules can help keep you happy and safe:

1 Limit how often you check your phone. (This is more difficult than it sounds.)

2 Leave your phone in the kitchen when you go to bed.

3 Don't look at your phone while crossing roads.

4 Know and follow the rules about cyberbullying (see page 122).

5 Ask an adult to help you block numbers of people who send you mean messages.

6 Don't answer calls from numbers you don't recognize. Let them go to voicemail.

7 Never give your mobile number to someone you don't know.

8 Never send pictures to someone you don't know.

9 If your parents call or text, always reply.

DEALING WITH BULLYING

Bullying is when someone keeps trying to hurt you. The person bullying you will sense that they have power over you and will make your life miserable. A one-off bit of nastiness is not bullying, even though it may be hurtful.

Bullying can happen in and out of school, and it happens to loads of young people. These are some of the things that bullies do:

- ⭐ Call you names.
- ⭐ Get you into trouble.
- ⭐ Hurt you by hitting, hair pulling, or other forms of violence.
- ⭐ Steal, hide, or damage your things.
- ⭐ Steal your money.
- ⭐ Turn your friends against you.
- ⭐ Spread rumors about you.
- ⭐ Taunt you.
- ⭐ Exclude you.
- ⭐ Make threats.
- ⭐ Post insulting messages, photos, or rumors on social media.
- ⭐ Send you nasty texts.

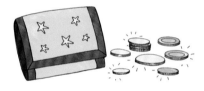

I am being bullied at school. What can I do?

If you are being bullied by other people at school, here are some suggestions for what you can do:

1 **You must tell someone:** It's not always easy to talk about it, but remember: it is never your fault that you are being bullied. Talk to your parents first. You may be able to sort out the problem yourself with your parents' support. If not, your school will have an anti-bullying policy and will take you seriously.

2 **You must try to make the bully realize that he or she does not have any power over you:** This is hard and you will need to pretend to be strong when you are feeling scared inside. First rule: never try to hit back or get into a fight; instead, face up to the bullies. When they start to taunt you, try to look confident. Stand at a normal distance from them and look them in the eye. Keep your voice calm and tell them to stop whatever they are doing. If you can, make a joke about it. Practice at home with your parents first.

3 **Keep away from the bullies:** Try to avoid places where they hang out. Stay near adults and other young people. Most bullying takes place where adults can't see you. Sit near the driver on the bus. Stay close to the teachers on duty. Spend time with real friends in and out of school.

4 **Talk to an expert:** Ring one of the helplines (see page 140).

For advice on what to do about cyberbullying (online), see page 122.

> If you feel you can't speak to the bullies, try to look confident as you walk past them. Keep your head up and look straight ahead. Wear headphones and pretend not to hear what they say. This is not easy either, so practice at home.

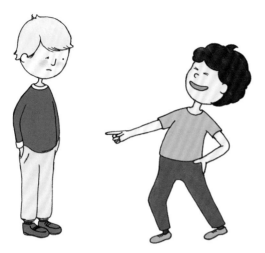

Other young people may bully you by laughing at you or calling you names. They may even hurt you physically. Remember: if this is happening to you, it is important to tell someone about it so that they can help you.

How are other people involved when someone is bullied?

When bullying is going on, all these people are involved:

The bully: Bullies often have problems in their own lives. They want to seem strong and get attention.

The person being bullied: Bullies like to bully people who are different in some way. Any excuse will do (e.g. wearing what they consider to be uncool clothes).

People who help and encourage the bully and may join in: They may be part of a bully's clique (see page 99).

People who watch and do nothing: They may laugh at what is going on and give the bully an audience.

People who don't watch or join in, but don't try to help: They know what's going on, but don't know what to do or are too scared to help.

People who support the person being bullied: They may confront the bully, get help, or simply comfort the person being bullied, showing their friendship.

 ## My friend is being bullied. What can I do?

Look at the list above and try to decide where you fit in? Now, whatever you did before, think whether you are strong enough to start becoming the person who fits the last description. Can you say to the bully, "That's a really mean thing to say. I don't know why you think you're so clever saying it?" Or find other put-downs? Can you say to your friend, "Don't take any notice of them. I'm still your friend"?

I've been bullying someone and now I feel bad about it. What can I do?

Young people can be mean. Few young people can say they've never hurt anyone or joined in bullying behavior, but if you have begun to understand how bad the person you've bullied feels, you've taken the first step away from bullying. Now, be brave and talk to an adult you trust. You may have bullied others because of your own problems. An adult can ensure you get help with these problems or just support you to stop the bullying (see page 118). Finally, although it's hard, apologize to the person you've bullied. They will feel safer and you will feel better.

Are adults allowed to hurt children?

If you are being hurt by an adult, it is not alright:

⭐ Adults should never deliberately hurt you physically by slapping, punching, kicking, hair pulling, or anything else. If you are smacked as a punishment (this is against the law in many countries), it should never be so hard that you are left with bruises, or happen so often that you are frightened to be at home.

⭐ Adults should not keep criticizing you, putting you down, or shouting at you so that you feel scared and miserable at home.

⭐ Adults should not neglect you. They must give you food to eat, clean clothes to wear, and a safe place to live with safe people who care for you.

⭐ Adults should not touch you in a way that makes you feel uncomfortable (see page 127).

If any of these things is happening to you, you must talk to someone who can help (see page 140 for a list of helpful organizations). Try to keep a diary, as this will help you explain what's going on.

WHAT IS CYBERBULLYING?

Cyberbullying can be even worse than other types of bullying because the bullies can reach you 24/7, so you are not even safe at home. It is also permanent. Spoken words are forgotten; stuff online can stay there forever.

Cyberbullies can hurt you in lots of different ways and the bullying can happen in text messages and on social media or gaming sites. They can make you very worried and depressed. These are some of the things they may do:

★ Write mean things about you or to you.

★ Post unkind rumors about you.

★ Threaten you.

★ Post mean or embarrassing images of you.

★ Exclude you from conversations and arrangements.

★ Use fake accounts so you don't know who is being mean to you.

★ Trick you into trusting them, so you share secrets and then they share those secrets.

★ Log into your account, pretend to be you, and post things you would never say.

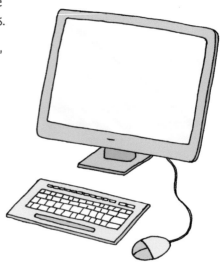

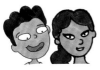

What should I do if I get a mean message?

If you get a mean message, follow these rules:

⭐ Do not send a mean message back. That's what the cyberbully wants you to do.

⭐ Do not reply at all.

⭐ Save the message and write down the date and time you got it.

⭐ One mean message is nasty, but it is probably not cyberbullying. Repeated meanness from the same person or group of people is, and you must report it.

If you are being cyberbullied, you must get help from an adult you trust. This is not something you can sort out on your own.

My friend is being cyberbullied. What should I do?

If you see a friend is being bullied online, try helping in these ways:

⭐ **Don't join in the bullying:** Don't "like," share, or comment on a mean post and don't forward mean texts to others.

⭐ **Write something yourself, but don't be mean, as that would make you into a bully:** Write something clear and calm. Say that what the bully is doing is hurtful and wrong. You could ask an adult to help you write your post.

⭐ **Support the person who was bullied:** Message them to let them know you like them and support them. Post positive things about them and your friendship.

⭐ **Report it:** Some social media sites have a "report it" button which lets you highlight anything you think shouldn't be there. It will be checked out, and the image or text can be removed.

DEALING WITH THE ONLINE WORLD

The internet is a brilliant place for finding out information, enjoying music, games, and videos, and keeping you connected with your friends, but there are not many police or laws there to keep you safe. Many social media sites don't let you have accounts until you are 13, but lots of young people get around this rule and, if you do, you are in more danger.

How do I keep safe online?

Just by accident, you can let horrible people know all about you, get friendly with people who are not who they say they are, send out embarrassing photos that the whole world can see, become a victim of cyberbullying (see page 122), let viruses into your computer, or find you are looking at pictures or websites that upset you. To keep you safe, your parents should install filters or monitoring software, and check that your privacy settings on social networks are as high as possible. Never download new apps or software without a parent's permission. When you are online (whether on a computer, tablet, smart phone, or games console), always keep to the following rules:

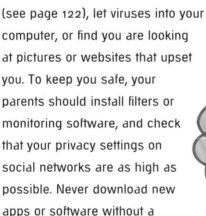

Talk to your parents about what you do online and show them websites or videos you like. If you talk to them, they will trust you more and allow you more privacy.

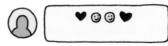

1 **Never post details about who you are:** This includes your full name, address, email address, mobile number, and the name of your school or clubs you go to, or any of your family's details.

2 **Never share your location.**

3 **Be careful about posting a picture or video of yourself:** Think (a) Would you be happy for all your friends and their friends and thousands of other people to see it? (b) Does the photo/video give away hidden information, such as your school logo/street sign/house number?

4 **Live streaming should only be to friends and followers:** Be careful what you say/do/show because the recording doesn't go away when you finish.

5 **Never tell anyone your passwords:** Your parents should know your passwords, but no one else, not even friends.

6 **Remember that not everyone online is who they say they are:** Strangers are more dangerous online because you can't see them. Adults can pretend to be children, boys to be girls, or girls to be boys.

7 **Don't believe everything you read or hear online:** There are a lot of liars out there and people trying to sell you things or get you to do things that are wrong. Celebrity vloggers are paid to advertise things they would never buy or use themselves.

8 **Don't "friend" people you don't know:** You are inviting them into your life and they may not be nice.

9 **Never arrange to meet someone you've met online without your parent's permission:** The person may not be who they say they are. If your parents agree to a meeting, you must take an adult with you.

10 **Switch off and tell if you don't like what you see:** If you see something online that makes you feel uncomfortable, unsafe, or worried, switch off and tell your parents immediately.

I've seen pictures about sex on my computer/phone. What are they?

Some adults post photos and videos of people having sex. This is called pornography. The sex is between actors. It isn't part of a loving relationship and often shows people doing things to each other which most real couples don't do when they make love. Women are often made to do what men want, rather than being equal. The actors' bodies are also made to look better than normal people's bodies. Seeing the images can make you feel uncomfortable and upset. These images can harm you at a time when you're first learning about sex. You may think, "This is what sex is like and I'll have to behave in those ways and look like those people and my partner will behave like that too." This is not true. Pornography is acting.

You may come across pornography by accident. If it comes up on your computer or phone, tell your parents so they can check the security settings. Alternatively, other young people may show you pornography and put pressure on you to watch it. They think it is a cool or grown-up thing to do and also a way to find out more about sex. Boys are more likely to do this than girls, but it can happen to both.

> Remember that pornography is not real sex and point this out to others. If someone is showing you images, walk away and, if you are worried, try to talk about it to a parent or trusted adult.

SOMEONE TRIED TO TOUCH ME IN A WAY I DIDN'T LIKE

Some adults can do nasty things to children and young people. They can start off seeming nice, but they don't really care about you. So, if someone touches you and something about the touch feels wrong, never put up with it. If you're not sure, follow these rules:

1 **Your body is your own:** It's not okay for anyone (not mom, dad, aunts, uncles, teachers, or friends) to touch you in a way that makes you feel uncomfortable.

2 **Privates are private:** Privates are all the parts covered by your swimwear and no one should ever touch you in these places, even as part of a game and even if it feels nice.

3 **No means No:** No one should try to persuade you (with pleading, presents, or threats) to let them touch you, or to make you touch them, in ways that make you uncomfortable.

4 **Secrets are suspicious:** Secrets should only be about good things like presents. People who touch you, and want to keep those touches a secret, know they're doing something bad.

5 **Talk to someone you trust:** Uncomfortable touches can come from someone you know well, even from someone in your family. Then it is difficult to know who to talk to and you may be scared about getting the person into trouble. A teacher or counselor in your school will know how to help you or you can call one of the helplines on page 140. You will always be listened to.

If an adult tries to get friendly by buying you gifts or encourages you to do things you know are wrong, be suspicious. They may be trying to gain your trust so they can do bad things to you. They may even make friends with your parents, so that they won't suspect. This is called grooming. Grooming can happen online, so always take an adult if you meet up with an online friend.

CHAPTER 8

MAKING BABIES AND FAMILIES

The reason why all the changes happen to your body is so that one day, when you are properly adult, you can choose to have a baby of your own. This chapter answers the questions you may have been embarrassed to ask about sex and how it can lead to the birth of a baby. It also tells you about genes and why you look like your parents and, because all babies need families, it tells you something about different kinds of families.

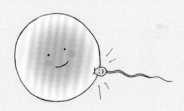

WHAT HAPPENS IN SEX AND PREGNANCY?

During puberty your hormones change so that as you get older, you have sexual feelings that make you want to be physically close to someone.

What happens when a man and woman have sex?

When a man and woman have sex, they first hug and kiss and stroke each other—usually when they are in bed together. The man's penis becomes erect (see page 66) and becomes the perfect size and shape to fit inside the woman's vagina. The vagina becomes wet and slippery. If the man and woman are naked, the penis can slip easily inside the vagina. One or both of them move so that the penis slides up and down in the vagina. This feels good for both of them and the feeling keeps getting stronger until the man has an orgasm and ejaculates (see page 69) semen inside the vagina. The woman can have an orgasm too (see page 53), but without the semen. Having sex is often called "making love" as it is one way that two people show their love for one another. Same-sex couples have different ways of making love.

So what has sex got to do with babies?

To make a baby, a sperm has to meet an egg. When a man and woman make love, millions of sperm are squirted into the vagina. Sperm are much too small to see. Under a microscope, they look a bit like tadpoles with tails. They use their tails to swim up through the uterus (womb) to the fallopian tubes. If there is an egg there, just one sperm will fertilize it, pushing inside its outer skin. Together the sperm and egg form the microscopic beginning of a baby.

How does a baby come from an egg and a sperm?

The fertilized egg travels along the fallopian tube and
into the uterus (womb) where it attaches to the
womb wall. From the moment it is fertilized, the
egg cell starts dividing: first into two cells, then
four, then eight, and so on. The ball of cells develops
into a baby according to the plan held in its genes (see
page 133). These are a combination of genes from its mom and its
dad. That's why a baby ends up looking like its mom in some ways
and its dad in others.

The baby is attached to the mother by a tube called the umbilical
cord. Everything the baby needs to live and grow comes from the
mother through the umbilical cord. The baby is tiny at first. It doesn't
look like a baby at all, and from the outside you can't tell that the
mother is pregnant. It takes about 40 weeks for the fertilized egg to
become a baby ready to be born
and by that time the mother's
tummy is huge! The baby is well
protected inside the womb
by a bag of liquid called the
amniotic sac, which stops
it getting banged and
bumped around.

Sometimes babies are
premature, which means they
are born too early. Then they
are much smaller and may have
to spend time in a heated cot
called an incubator, with tubes
to help them breathe.

Do you always make a baby when you have sex?

No, but when a man and woman have sex there is always the chance that the woman could become pregnant and there is no way of knowing when it will happen. Most couples like to make love, but they do not want very large families, so they use contraception to stop the woman getting pregnant. There are lots of different types of contraception such as a pill that a woman takes every day to stop her eggs being released or a condom which fits over a man's penis to stop sperm getting into the woman. If they decide that it's the right time for them to have a baby, they stop using contraception.

Now that I have started my periods, could I have a baby?

Yes, you could get pregnant and a boy who has started producing sperm could become a father, but you're not yet adult enough to have sex or bring up a baby. Sex should be part of a loving relationship and you aren't ready for that. Having sex when you're too young can leave you feeling hurt and upset. In many countries it is illegal for children your age to have sex, even if they've gone through puberty.

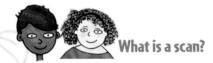

What is a scan?

A scan is a video made by a machine called an ultrasound which uses sound and echoes to show the baby inside the mother's uterus (womb) before it is born. If someone you know is pregnant, they may show you a photo from their scan. They might also let you feel the baby moving inside their tummy. Doctors use scans to check how big the baby is, if it is healthy, and if the mother is going to have twins. They can also see if the baby is a boy or girl. Some parents like to know this before their baby is born; others prefer it to be a surprise.

WHAT IS A GENE?

How often have people said to you, "You look just like your dad (or mom)!" That's because they've passed their genes on to you. Your genes are a bit like a computer program for building you. They say what color your eyes are, how you smile, how tall you are, whether you are musical or athletic, and a lot more. Genes are arranged on chromosomes. These are tiny, spaghetti-like structures which come in pairs and are found in nearly every cell in your body.

There are 23 pairs of chromosomes in each cell, making 46 in total. However, in sperm and eggs, there are only 23 single chromosomes. When a sperm fertilizes an egg to make a baby, the two sets of chromosomes join, so you inherit features from your mom and dad. One special chromosome comes in two different forms, known as X and Y. When an X chromosome meets a Y chromosome, the baby is a boy. If two X chromosomes join, it's a girl. Chromosomes and genes are made of DNA (deoxyribonucleic acid). To find out more, check out the websites on page 141.

Remember, though, that as well as your genes your actions are very important in making you who you are. You can't change how tall you are, but genes don't give you an excuse not to practice if you want to be a good musician or athlete!

WHAT HAPPENS WHEN A BABY IS BORN?

You have all seen pregnant women with tummies so big they look like they are about to pop, but how do babies actually get out of their mothers' tummies?

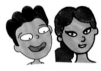 ## How is a baby born?

When the baby is ready to be born the uterus (womb) begins to squeeze. The mother feels the squeezes (called contractions) and knows that she has "gone into labor." This means her body is beginning to push the baby out. It's called labor because it is hard work and often takes quite a long time. The baby is pushed out, head first, through the opening at the bottom of the womb and the vagina. This is what happens when the baby is born:

⭐ The head comes through first because the head is the biggest part.

⭐ When the head appears between the mother's legs, a midwife or doctor helps pull the baby out gently.

⭐ The first thing a baby does when it is born is cry. This fills its lungs with air.

⭐ The midwife lays the baby on the mother's tummy and cuts the umbilical cord. Your tummy button is the scar where your umbilical cord was cut when you were born.

⭐ The mother cradles her baby and it often has its first feed from the mother's breast.

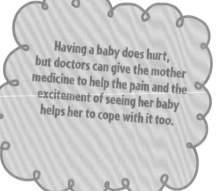

Having a baby does hurt, but doctors can give the mother medicine to help the pain and the excitement of seeing her baby helps her to cope with it too.

My mom has a scar on her tummy from where I was born. Why wasn't I born through her vagina?

If doctors think it might be difficult for the mother to push her baby out safely, they do an operation called a Cesarean section. They cut a small hole in the mother's tummy and lift the baby out. Many babies are born in this way. There are lots of reasons why. For example, the baby might be the wrong way round, so it would come out feet first, or it might be very big.

How do twins happen?

Sometimes when the fertilized egg splits into two, it splits right apart and each half becomes the beginning of a baby. These are identical twins. They are always the same sex and look exactly the same. Non-identical twins happen when two eggs are released by the ovary at the same time and are fertilized by two different sperm, and each egg becomes a baby. These twins may be a boy and a girl, two boys, or two girls, and they will look completely different, just like any brothers and sisters look different.

Occasionally, a woman has triplets (three babies), quadruplets (four babies), or even more. Because there is not much space for two or more babies in the womb, twins and triplets are often smaller when they are born and are also more likely to be born by Cesarean section.

THERE ARE ALL SORTS OF FAMILIES

How many people are there in your family? Do you know families that are very different from yours? Families are really important for bringing up children, but every family is different and has its own strengths and weaknesses.

 ## Does a baby always need a mom and dad?

For a baby to grow up happy and healthy it needs to be brought up in a family that loves and cares for it. Looking after a baby is not easy. You are responsible for it every minute of every day. The baby grows into a child, and then into an adult, and you are still responsible for it. Bringing up children is hard work (and very expensive), so having a baby is an important decision. Every baby comes from an egg and a sperm; that doesn't mean, however, that every child lives with a mom and a dad. There are lots of different types of families. Here are some of them:

Nuclear families: Mom and dad and one or more children.

Single-parent families: One mom/ dad and one or more children.

Extended families: Mom, dad, grandparents, children, aunts or uncles all living together in one house.

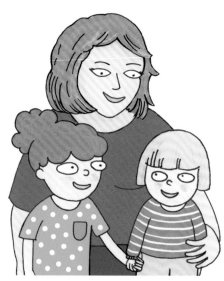

Same-sex families: Two moms and one or more children or two dads and one or more children.

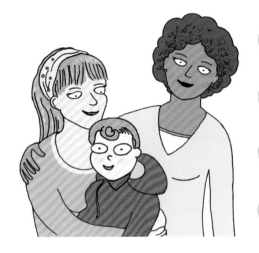

Childless couples: Couples with no children, either because they didn't want any or because, for medical reasons, the woman doesn't get pregnant.

Blended families (mom, step-dad + children + dad, step-mom): Children whose parents have separated may have two different families and spend time with each. If their parents have new partners, they may also have step-brothers and step-sisters in those families. If their mom or dad has another baby with their new partner, the baby will be their half-brother or half-sister.

Foster families: These are families who care for children when their own family can't look after them. It could be for a long time or just for a few weeks, but it isn't permanent.

Adopted children: Some families may adopt a child or children whose families cannot look after them. This isn't like a foster family because adoption is forever. Many adopted children know who their birth parents are. They may send letters to them and perhaps meet them.

My friend says she was an IVF baby. What does this mean?

Sometimes a man and woman want a baby, but can't get pregnant. This is due to medical reasons in the man and/or woman. Then eggs can be taken from one of the woman's ovaries and put together with some sperm in a "test tube" in a laboratory. The embryo (the very early stage of a baby) is put back in the woman's uterus (womb) and she can have a normal pregnancy. This is called in-vitro fertilization (IVF). Sadly, it doesn't always work.

How do gay couples have children?

It can be harder for gay couples (two men or two women) to have children. They can choose to adopt a child, but they often want a baby that has some of their genes (see page 133). Two men can find a woman who is happy to have a baby for them. The woman becomes pregnant with sperm from one of the men. When she has the baby she gives it to the men. A woman who does this is called a surrogate mother. Two women can have sperm from a sperm bank put into one

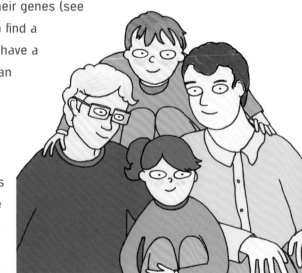

of them, so she becomes pregnant. (Some men donate sperm to be kept in a sperm bank, just like adults can donate blood.)

My parents are separating/getting divorced. What can I do?

Sadly many parents decide to separate or divorce (the legal ending of a marriage) because they feel they can no longer live together. This can be for lots of reasons, but you should never feel that it is your fault or that you can do anything to change it. Remember: they are divorcing each other, not you, and they will both still love you when they are apart. You may feel lots of strong emotions, including huge sadness that your family is breaking up, anger with your parents for causing the change, fear and confusion about what will happen next, or perhaps relief that the arguments will stop and life at home will become more peaceful. Your parents are likely to be stressed and upset, too. Talking to them about what is going on can be helpful. They may not have all the answers to your questions, but it is better that they understand how you are feeling. Try to help them by not having arguments and lending a hand at home. It is useful to talk to other adults or friends you can trust, or call a helpline (see page 140) if necessary. Don't try to cope with this on your own.

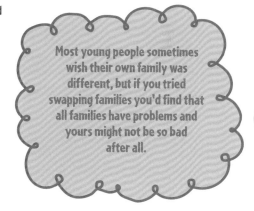

Most young people sometimes wish their own family was different, but if you tried swapping families you'd find that all families have problems and yours might not be so bad after all.

FIND OUT MORE

Helplines

When you don't know who to talk to about something that is worrying you, call one of the following numbers. No issue is too small for them to help you with.

You can call 24/7, and the calls are free and confidential (which means they won't tell anybody about your call, unless you or somebody else is in danger).

Alternatively, you can go to the organization's website to find other ways of contacting them and for loads of other useful information and advice.

If you live in the USA, call **Boys Town** (a helpline for girls and boys) on 1-800-448-3000 or go to http://www.yourlifeyourvoice.org/Pages/home.aspx (or call Childhelp on 1-800-422-4453)

If you live in the UK, call **Childline** on 0800 1111 or go to www.childline.org.uk

If you live in Australia, call **Kidshelpline** on 1800 55 1850 or go to https://kidshelpline.com.au/

If you live in Canada, call **Kids Help Phone** on 1-800-668-6868 or go to https://kidshelpphone.ca

Further information

All the organizations with helplines have websites with much more information than we have room for in this book. Other useful websites:

http://www.cyh.com/SubDefault.aspx?p=255
Kids' Health, an excellent Australian website especially for kids

https://kidshealth.org/en/kids/grow/
Kidshealth, an American website, with sections for kids and parents

www.nhs.uk/Livewell/puberty/Documents/fpa-periods-PDF.pdf
Periods: What you need to know (this is a PDF which you could print off)

YouTube videos

Inside Puberty (this series also has separate videos for boys and girls)
https://www.youtube.com/watch?v=Rsj6dW6qKRc
What is DNA and How Does it Work?
https://www.youtube.com/watch?v=zwibgNGe4aY
What is a chromosome?
https://www.youtube.com/watch?v=IePMXxQ-KWY

Pregnancy

Fetal development: https://www.babycentre.co.uk/pregnancy-week-by-week
and https://www.youtube.com/watch?v=WtDknjng8TA

This website and video have been made for pregnant women, but are very
good for seeing images of how a baby develops in the uterus (womb) week
by week. If your mom or someone else you know is pregnant, it is interesting
to see just what the baby looks like at each stage of their pregnancy.

Help for parents and carers

Being a parent or carer isn't always easy. These websites offer advice
on looking after children.

https://childmind.org/article/10-tips-for-parenting-your-pre-teen/
https://learning.nspcc.org.uk/media/1195/positive-parenting.pdf
https://www.mermaidsuk.org.uk Mermaids, providing family and individual
support for gender diverse and transgender children and young people.
https://www.nspcc.org.uk/preventing-abuse/keeping-children-safe/
talking-about-difficult-topics/
https://youngminds.org.uk

ABOUT THE CONSULTANTS

Dr Frances Butcher (BMBS MA MSc MFPH) is a doctor specializing in public health. After several years working in clinical medicine, she now looks at health from a population perspective and has worked in various organizations, including Public Health England, NHS England, and the University of Oxford. A priority for her work is the prevention of ill health from an early age, as improving children's physical and mental health, alongside their social wellbeing, is key to maximizing their life opportunities in adulthood.

Dr Rosanna Bevan (BSc BMBS MRCPCH) is a doctor working in mental health, who formerly worked as a pediatrician. She is also a volunteer youth worker who works with trans and gender-variant young people and has wide experience of the problems young people face at puberty. She has done research in children's sleep and has worked with the Royal College of Paediatrics and Child Health on making training for pediatric doctors more inclusive of gay, lesbian, bisexual, and trans young people.

James Hull (BA Hons PGCE) has worked in education for 10 years, blending teaching and pastoral care in outdoor education centers, schools, and colleges. He spent five years as a houseparent in a boarding school, working with children of 8 years and above, and has also worked as chief instructor at an activity center running residential activity courses. As such, he has plenty of experience of dealing with the practical problems, emotional needs, and safety of both boys and girls who are going through puberty.

INDEX

ACKNOWLEDGMENTS

*With thanks to the children and their parents who provided
useful feedback on the content and look of the book;
the consultants for their invaluable input; and to Caroline West,
my editor, for helping to pull the book into shape.*